T0076121

TUMOR SUPPRESSOR GENES
IN BREAST CANCER

TUMOR SUPPRESSOR GENES IN BREAST CANCER

MARC LACROIX

Nova Biomedical Publishers, Inc.
New York

Copyright © 2008 by Nova Science Publishers, Inc.

All rights reserved. No part of this book may be reproduced, stored in a retrieval system or transmitted in any form or by any means: electronic, electrostatic, magnetic, tape, mechanical photocopying, recording or otherwise without the written permission of the Publisher.

For permission to use material from this book please contact us:
Telephone 631-231-7269; Fax 631-231-8175
Web Site: http://www.novapublishers.com

NOTICE TO THE READER

The Publisher has taken reasonable care in the preparation of this book, but makes no expressed or implied warranty of any kind and assumes no responsibility for any errors or omissions. No liability is assumed for incidental or consequential damages in connection with or arising out of information contained in this book. The Publisher shall not be liable for any special, consequential, or exemplary damages resulting, in whole or in part, from the readers' use of, or reliance upon, this material.

Independent verification should be sought for any data, advice or recommendations contained in this book. In addition, no responsibility is assumed by the publisher for any injury and/or damage to persons or property arising from any methods, products, instructions, ideas or otherwise contained in this publication.

This publication is designed to provide accurate and authoritative information with regard to the subject matter covered herein. It is sold with the clear understanding that the Publisher is not engaged in rendering legal or any other professional services. If legal or any other expert assistance is required, the services of a competent person should be sought. FROM A DECLARATION OF PARTICIPANTS JOINTLY ADOPTED BY A COMMITTEE OF THE AMERICAN BAR ASSOCIATION AND A COMMITTEE OF PUBLISHERS.

LIBRARY OF CONGRESS CATALOGING-IN-PUBLICATION DATA

Tumor suppressor genes in breast cancer / Marc Lacroix, editor.
    p. ; cm.
  Includes bibliographical references and index.
  ISBN 978-1-60456-326-9 (softcover)
  1. Breast--Cancer--Genetic aspects. 2. Antioncogenes. I. Lacroix, Marc, 1963-
  [DNLM: 1. Breast Neoplasms--genetics. 2. Genes, Tumor Suppressor. WP 870 T9256 2008]
RC280.B8T865 2008
616.99'449042--dc22
                         2007049392

Published by Nova Science Publishers, Inc. ✛ New York

CONTENTS

Preface   vii

Abbreviations   ix

Chapter 1   Introduction   1

Chapter 2   Inactivating Events:
                    LOH, Point Mutations,Methylation   3

Chapter 3   TP53: A Major TSG in (Breast) Cancer   5

Chapter 4   BRCA1 and BRCA2,
                    Major TSGs in Familial Breast Cancer   9

Chapter 5   Detailed Information on Candidate TSGs   11

Chapter 6   Conclusion   67

Acknowledgments   69

References   71

Index   103

PREFACE

Breast cancer is characterized by the accumulation of genetic alterations, including point mutations and loss of entire DNA regions ("loss of heterozygosity" or LOH). Among genes that are affected by such events, the "tumor suppressor genes" (TSGs) have a peculiar interest since they often occupy pivotal positions in regulatory networks that control the cell cycle and/or encompass various signal transduction cascades. While a number of genes have been suggested as candidate TSGs in breast cancer, only a few of them have been confirmed in this status. They include TP53, BRCA1, BRCA2 and are mainly involved in the control of DNA repair, cell proliferation, apoptosis and signaling. Some TSGs are linked to familial (hereditary) forms of breast cancer. The exact definition of what is a TSG is still debated. Recently, genes not affected by mutation or even LOH, but occasionally methylated, have been considered as TSGs.

ABBREVIATIONS

DSB	double-strand breaks;
GC	gene conversion;
HR	homology-directed recombination;
LOH	loss of heterozygosity;
NER	nucleotide-excision repair;
NHEJ	non-homologous end joining;
SSA	single-strand annealing;
TSG	tumor suppressor gene.

Chapter 1

INTRODUCTION

Breast cancer is not an organ, nor a cell disease: it is a genetic disease. Indeed, it is well accepted that a series of genetic changes must occur for normal mammary epithelial cells to transform themselves into breast cancer cells. Changes associated with malignant transformation of cells occur on two types of genes, namely "oncogenes" and "tumor suppressor genes" (TSGs). The abnormal activity of oncogenes has been well described as one possible mechanism to transform normal cells. This activity may result from point mutations, gene amplification, or chromosomal translocations. The inactivation of TSGs, which normally prevent the onset of a cancer, "classically" involves point mutations or chromosomal deletions. More recently, additional mechanisms have been proposed such as gene promoter methylation (epigenetic modification).

Both oncogenes and TSGs do much more than just stimulate or prevent, respectively, the onset of a cancer. They are tightly interwoven. They are intimately involved in the regulation of fundamental processes affecting almost every aspect of normal cell growth, differentiation, and cell death. Like oncogenes, TSGs occupy pivotal positions in regulatory networks that encompass various signal transduction cascades. Therefore, these pathways often involve an interaction of different TSGs. Thus, it is often difficult to associate breast cancers with one specific TSG. However, a minority of breast tumors (5-10%) has a hereditary origin and is clearly associated to inherited mutations in well-defined TSGs: BRCA1, BRCA2, TP53, ATM, CHEK2, PTEN, TP53, STK11...

Chapter 2

INACTIVATING EVENTS:
LOH, POINT MUTATIONS, METHYLATION

TSGs are considered to act mostly in a recessive fashion, i.e. some abnormality must affect both gene alleles. According to the classical 'two-hit' hypothesis proposed by Knudson (1971), inactivation of TSGs is caused by TSG deletion due to chromosomal loss of one allele, and mutation of the other remaining allele (the order of events is still unknown, see Wilentz *et al.* 2001). Recently, the Knudson's model was extended to include epigenetically inactivated genes, mainly by hypermethylation (see notably Kopelovich *et al.* 2003, Esteller 2005). In such cases, the first "hit" is the genetic knockout of one allele and the second "hit" is promoter hypermethylation. It has even been suggested that for some TSGs, both alleles could be silenced by hypermethylation only, in total absence of LOH or point mutation. As compared to gene mutation, which is transmitted to daughter cells, the persistence of gene promoter hypermethylation during tumor progression is not warranted. It must be noted that a second event may be unnecessary for TSGs exhibiting haploinsufficiency, as notably suggested for PTEN in prostate cancer (Kwabi-Addo *et al.* 2001). Nonetheless, it is widely presumed that regions of consistently high LOH are functionally important in tumorigenesis.

Chromosomal loss is mostly analyzed by karyotypic studies or loss of heterozygosity (LOH) studies. Genome-wide maps of regions of LOH have been published (Kerangueven *et al.* 1997; Miller *et al.* 2003; Mao *et al.* 2005). Losses may also be detected by using comparative genomic hybridization, representational oligonucleotide microarray analysis (Lucito *et al.* 2003) or high-density oligonucleotide array-based SNP genotyping (Huang *et al.* 2004). Mutations in TSGs are most frequently studied by sequencing of the gene of interest or by single strand chain polymorphism analysis (SSCP). In many cases, mutations can result in truncated protein products which are easy to detect. Methylation of gene promoter may be analyzed by methylation-specific PCR (MSP) or bisulfite treatment-specific PCR (BSP).

Chapter 3

TP53: A Major TSG in (Breast) Cancer

TP53 encodes P53. This protein plays an important role in regulating cell fate in response to various stresses, either genotoxic (DNA alterations induced by irradiation, UV, carcinogens, cytotoxic drugs) or not (hypoxia, nucleotide depletion, oncogene activation, microtubule disruption, loss of normal cell contacts). It may be viewed as a node for the stress signals, which are then transduced, mainly through the ability of P53 to act as a transcription factor. P53 exerts its anti-proliferative action by inducing reversible or irreversible (senescence) cell cycle arrest, or apoptosis. It may also enhance DNA repair and inhibit angiogenesis. It is believed that the tumor suppressing activity of P53 is exerted mainly through the triggering of apoptosis. Indeed, loss of P53 activity disrupts apoptosis and accelerates the appearance of tumors in transgenic mice, which generally succumb before reaching the age of 1 year. In non-stress conditions, the nuclear level of wild-type P53 is kept low, as the protein is labeled for degradation by the ubiquitin ligase MDM2 (t½ for P53 = 20-40 min). In stress conditions, P53 is modified through phosphorylation, cis/trans isomerization, acetylation, methylation, sumoylation, neddylation and/or glycosylation at multiple sites, which prevents its interaction with MDM2 and allows its accumulation (Lacroix *et al.* 2006).

TP53 is located at 17p13.1. Chromosome 17p is among the most frequently deleted regions in a variety of human malignancies including breast cancer. It has been found that 73% (37 of 51) of the breast tumors exhibit LOH at one or more loci at 17p13, and losses at 17p13 were seen more frequently in large and poorly differentiated tumors with high proliferative activity (Seitz *et al.* 2001). One of these loci is 17p13.1. Another frequently deleted locus, at 17p13.3, contains

HIC1, a target of P53 (Seitz *et al.* 2001, Britschgi *et al.* 2006). See below the discussion on HIC1.

TP53 mutations are the most frequent genetic events in human cancer. More than 21,000 mutations have been compiled by the International Agency for Research on Cancer (IARC, http://www-p53.iarc.fr/) (Olivier *et al.* 2002). They have been found in most types of tumors, with frequencies ranging from 5% (cervix) to 50% (lung). Since there is no evidence that TP53 lies in a hyper-mutable region of the genome, cells that have lost P53 function are likely to be selected during cancer development. The P53 function is often altered in breast cancer. Between 20 and 35% of breast tumors have been shown to express a mutant P53, and this percentage is even higher in a panel of widely-used breast cancer cell lines. The pattern and codon distributions of P53 mutations in breast tumors show a very similar profile to all other cancers, including similar hot spots. Indeed, 34% of P53 mutations affect only 10 residues – 175, 176, 179, 213, 220, 245, 248, 249, 273, and 282; three residues (175, 248 and 273) contribute 18% of mutations. More than 90% of all mutations affect the P53 central core region (residues 103–292), which interacts with DNA. To date, only 2% and 5% of all mutations have been located to non-central P53 regions 1–101 and 293–393 respectively (Lacroix *et al.* 2006).

Most TP53 mutations observed in breast cancer are of somatic origin. However, TP53 mutations may also be observed in the rare familial autosomal Li–Fraumeni syndrome. It is characterized by a high incidence of multiple early cancers, including breast tumors. Other hereditary breast cancers may be due to mutations in genes coding for P53 modulator proteins. A significant proportion of these cancers have been associated with mutations of BRCA1. BRCA1 may interact with P53 and has been viewed as a 'scaffold' for P53 response (Hohenstein and Giles 2003). Of interest, BRCA1 tumors often express TP53 mutations, but it remains to be established if this reflects the need for P53 inactivation for the development of BRCA1 tumors to occur, or rather if the loss of BRCA1-associated DNA repair properties may explain, at least partly, the high frequency of TP53 mutations (Lacroix and Leclercq, 2005).

Other mutations leading to familial syndromes accompanied by a high occurrence of breast cancer may affect BRCA2, ATM (Ataxia-Telangiectasia), CHEK2 (Li-Fraumeni-like syndrome), STK11 (Peutz-Jeghers syndrome), or PTEN (Cowden syndrome) (Lacroix and Leclercq 2005). The products of two of these genes, ATM and CHEK2, are involved in P53 activation, while the product of PTEN increases P53 activity by antagonizing the cell survival effects mediated by the AKT-MDM2 pathway (see above). A physical interaction between STK11 and P53 has been reported and STK11 appears to regulate specific P53-dependent growth-suppression and apoptosis pathways (Karuman *et al.* 2001). It also seems that mutations of TP53 and STK11 cooperate in the acceleration of tumorigenesis (Wei *et al.* 2005).

In cells expressing a mutant P53, this protein is generally no longer able to control cell proliferation, which results in inefficient DNA repair and genetic instability. In fact, the great majority of mutant P53 is defective in transactivation and may exert a dominant negative effect by preventing wild-type P53 from binding to the promoter of its target genes. When introduced into cells expressing a wild-type P53, a mutant P53 can transform and give to these cells a more aggressive phenotype. This is aggravated by the fact that mutated P53 may accumulate since it can no longer be ubiquitinated by MDM2.

From a clinical point of view, P53 mutations, particularly those affecting the DNA binding core regions, are generally associated with tumor cell resistance to chemotherapeutic drugs, with the notable exception of mitotic spindle poisons.

Significantly, amplification of the MDM2 gene is observed in a significant fraction of most common human sarcomas.

The importance of P53 in cell death and the high frequency of mutations affecting this protein have generated a significant interest in exploiting the P53 pathway for novel cancer therapies. Various approaches have been exploited. Probably the most promising involves small compounds used for the restoration of P53 function to lesions that carry full-length P53 protein with one amino acid change in the DNA-binding core domain. In theory, such compounds should only have an effect on cancer cells, because the core domain of wild-type P53 in normal cells is already structurally intact. Ellipticine (5,11-dimethyl-6H-pyrido[4,3-b]carbazole), the styrylquinazoline CP-31398, and PRIMA-1 (2,2-Bis(hy-droxymethyl)-1-azabicyclo[2,2,2]octan-3-one) have been shown to restore function to a subset of P53 mutants. PRIMA-1 (for P53 reactivation and induction of massive apoptosis-1) may synergize with chemotherapy (cisplatin) in inducing apoptosis in tumors, indicating the potential advantage of combined therapies. Screening of a chemical library identified another small molecule named RITA (for reactivation of P53 and induction of tumor cell apoptosis). It prevents P53-MDM2 interaction in vitro and in vivo and has anti-tumor activity. The maleimide-derived molecule, MIRA-1, can reactivate DNA binding and preserve the active conformation of mutant P53 protein in vitro and restore transcriptional transactivation to mutant P53 in living cells. The structural analogue MIRA-3 shows anti-tumor activity in vivo against human mutant P53-carrying tumor xenografts in SCID mice (Lacroix *et al.* 2006).

Chapter 4

BRCA1 AND BRCA2, MAJOR TSGS IN FAMILIAL BREAST CANCER

In a series of 127 breast carcinomas, LOH was found in the BRCA1 and BRCA2 regions in 49% and 44% of tumors, respectively (Gonzalez *et al.* 1999).

A family history of breast cancer is one of the most significant risk factors for the development of the disease. It is estimated that 5–10% of all breast carcinomas is inherited, the other 90–95% of cases being considered as "sporadic". The BRCA1 and BRCA2 genes account for autosomal dominant transmission of susceptibility in a majority of families with hereditary breast-ovarian (BRCA1/BRCA2) or male breast cancers (BRCA2). Detailed descriptions of the BRCA1 and BRCA2 genes, including the numerous distinct mutations that can alter the function of their corresponding protein, have been the subject of many reviews (see for instance Carter 2001; Borg 2001; Iau et al. 2001; Welcsh and King 2001; Starita and Parvin 2003; Rosen *et al.* 2003; Powell and Kachnic 2003; Lacroix and Perec 2003; Lacroix and Leclercq 2005; Lacroix and Leclercq 2006) and will not be further discussed here. Both BRCA1 and BRCA2 are long genes that may be targeted by hundreds of different mutations, of which many have been observed only once. Data on BRCA1 and BRCA2 mutations may be found in the Breast Information Core (http://research.nhgri. nih.gov/bic/) and Human Gene Mutation (http://archive.uwcm.ac.uk/uwcm/mg/hgmd0.html) databases.

The development of BRCA1 or BRCA2 tumors has been attributed mainly to the loss of the DNA repair function ensured by these proteins. The BRCA1 protein normally resides in a nuclear multiprotein complex, including BRCA2, BARD1, and RAD51, and the DNA damage repair proteins MSH2, MLH1, MSH6, ATM, NBS1, MRE11, RAD50, BLM, and RFC. This BRCA1-associated genome surveillance complex (BASC) functions as a sensor of abnormal DNA structures, such as double-strand breaks and base pair mismatches. BRCA1 has been suggested to have a pivotal function within BASC by coordinating the actions of damage-sensing proteins and executive repair proteins. BRCA1 may also act as a transcriptional regulator of genes involved. in checkpoint reinforcement and, in complexes with BARD1, as a ubiquitin ligase (reviewed in Carter 2001; Borg 2001; Iau *et al.* 2001; Welcsh and King 2001). Thus, mutations of BRCA1 likely impair the repair of damaged DNA, thereby rendering the mutant cells prone to malignant transformation.

Indeed, both BRCA1 and BRCA2 are involved in DNA double-strand breaks (DSB) repair. In eukaryotes, two major pathways exist to repair DSB: non-homologous end joining (NHEJ) and homology-directed recombination (HR). NHEJ repairs adjacent broken DNA ends with little or no requirement for extensive sequence homology, whereas the more accurate HR requires an intact template of a homologous sequence either in a homologous chromosome or in a sister chromatid. HR may occur either by "gene conversion" (GC) or by an error-prone "single-strand annealing" (SSA) mechanism. BRCA2 is involved mainly, if not solely, in HR by GC, through its interaction with the essential DSB repair protein RAD51. BRCA1 mutations seem to impair both classes of HR, but BRCA1 is also possibly involved in NHEJ by a way implying its colocalization with the RAD50-MRE11-NBS1 complex. In addition to its importance in DSB repair, BRCA1 could also play some role in nucleotide-excision repair (NER). Thus, the implication in DNA repair appears to be greater for BRCA1 than for BRCA2. BRCA1 and BRCA2 must not be seen as single components of linear chains of molecules linking DNA alterations to DNA repair. It is increasingly recognized that they are members of complex and versatile protein network(s) involved in multiple functions. They have been associated to transcription transcription regulation and chromatin remodeling, cell cycle and centrosome regulation, apoptosis induction, ubiquitination and protein degradation.

Chapter 5

DETAILED INFORMATION ON CANDIDATE TSGS

Besides TP53, BRCA1 and BRCA2, a number of genes have been proposed as candidate TSGs. They are listed in Table 1 and further described below:

Table 1. A list of genes that have been proposed as candidate TSGs

OMIM	Gene name(s)	Name of encoded protein(s)
1p31-p22	CLCA2	Chloride channel, calcium-activated, 2
1p31	DIRAS3; ARHI; RHOI; NOEY2	DIRAS family, GTP-binding RAS-like 3; ras homolog gene family, member I; rho-related GTP-binding protein I; NOEY2 protein
1p31.1	LPHH1	Latrophilin homolog 1; lectomedin 1
1p31.3	TTC4	Tetratricopeptide repeat domain 4
1p32	RAD54L; RAD54	RAD54-like; RAD54
1p33-p31	FABP3; MDGI	Fatty acid binding protein 3; mammary-derived growth inhibitor
1p36	RUNX3; CBFA3; AML2	Runt-related transcription factor 3; core-binding factor, Runt domain, alpha subunit 3; AML2 protein
1p36	PRDM2(1); RIZ(1)	PR domain-containing protein 2, transcript 1; retinoblastoma protein-binding zinc finger protein, transcript 1
1p36.11	SFN; 14-3-3σ	Stratifin; 14-3-3σ protein
3p12	ROBO1; DUTT1	Roundabout, axon guidance receptor, homolog 1 (Drosophila); deleted in U Twenty Twenty
3p14.2	PTPG; PTPRG	Protein-tyrosine phosphatase, gamma; protein-tyrosine phosphatase, receptor-type, gamma

Table 1. (Continued)

OMIM	Gene name(s)	Name of encoded protein(s)
3p14.2	FHIT; FRA3B, included	Fragile histidine triad gene; fragile site 3p14.2, included; AP3A hydrolase
3p21	PB1; BAF180	Polybromo 1, chicken homolog of BRG1-associated factor, 180 kD; BRG1-associated factor, 180 kD
3p21.3	RASSF1(A)	Ras association (RalGDS/AF-6) domain family 1, transcript A
3p21.3	RBM5; LUCA-15; H37	RNA binding motif protein 5
3p21.3	TUSC4; NPRL2	Tumor suppressor candidate 4
3p21.3	TMEM158; RIS1	Transmembrane protein 158; Ras-induced senescence 1
3p21.3	SEMA3B	Sema domain, immunoglobulin domain (Ig), short basic domain, secreted, (semaphorin) 3B
3p22	TGFBR2; HNPCC6	Transforming growth factor, beta receptor II, 70-80kD; colorectal cancer, hereditary nonpolyposis, type 6
3p22.2	APRG1; C3orf35	AP20 region protein 1; chromosome 3 open reading frame 35
3p24	RARB(2)	Retinoic acid receptor, beta polypeptide, transcript 2
3p26-p25	VHL	Von Hippel Lindau gene
3q22-q24	ATR; FRP1	Ataxia telangiectasia and rad3-related; FRAP-related protein 1
4p15.2	SLIT2	Slit, Drosophila, homolog of, 2
4q25-q26	PRDM5	PR domain containing 5
4q34-q35	HPGD; PGDH1	NAD(+)-dependent 15-hydroxyprostaglandin dehydrogenase; 15-hydroxyprostaglandin dehydrogenase, type I
5p13	DAB2; C9	Disabled homolog 2, mitogen-responsive phosphoprotein (Drosophila); complement component-9
5q21-q22	APC	Adenomatosis polyposis coli
5q31.1	IRF1	Interferon regulatory factor 1
6q24	PLAGL1; ZAC; LOT1	Pleomorphic adenoma gene-like 1; ZAC tumor suppressor; lost on transformation 1
6q24-q25.1	LATS1; WARTS	LATS, large tumor suppressor, homolog 1 (Drosophila); warts gene
6q26	IGF2R; MPRI	Insulin-like growth factor II receptor; mannose-6-phosphate receptor; mannose-6-phosphate receptor, cation-independent
7q31.1-q31.2	ST7; TSG7; RAY1; FAM4A1; HELG	Suppression of tumorigenicity 7

OMIM	Gene name(s)	Name of encoded protein(s)
8p12-p11.1	SFRP1; FRP	Secreted frizzled-related protein 1; frizzled-related protein;
8p21	DLC1; ARHGAP7	Deleted in liver cancer 1; rho GTPase activating protein 7
8p21	BNIP3L	BCL2/adenovirus E1B 19-kD protein-interacting protein 3-like
8p21.2	RHOBTB2; DBC2	Rho-related BTB domain containing 2; deleted in breast cancer 2
8p22	LZTS1, FEZ1; F37	Leucine zipper, putative tumor suppressor 1
8p22	MTUS1; ATIP	Mitochondrial tumor suppressor 1; angiotensin II receptor-interacting protein
8p23	MCPH1; BRIT1	Microcephalin 1; BRCT-repeat inhibitor of TERT expression 1
8q11.2	ST18	Suppression of tumorigenicity 18
9p21	CDKN2A; $p16^{INK4A}$; $p14^{ARF}$	Cyclin-dependent kinase inhibitor 2A (p16, inhibits CDK4)
9q22	SYK	Spleen tyrosine kinase
9q33.1-q33.3	DAB2IP; AIP1	DAB2 interacting protein; ASK1-interacting protein
9q34	TSC1	Tuberous sclerosis 1; hamartin
10q23.31	PTEN; MMAC1	Phosphatase and tensin homolog; mutated in multiple advanced cancers 1
10q24	PDCD4	Programmed cell death 4
10q26	MGMT	Methylguanine-DNA methyltransferase
11p13	WT1	Wilms tumor-1
11p15.2-p15.1	TSG101	Tumor susceptibility gene 101
11p15.5	CDKN1C; BWS	Cyclin-dependent kinase inhibitor 1C (p57, Kip2); Beckwith-Wiedemann syndrome
11q13	CST6	Cystatin-M
11q21-q24	IGSF4; TSLC1; ST17; NECL2	Immunoglobulin superfamily, member 4; tumor suppressor in lung cancer; suppression of tumorigenicity 17; nectin-like protein 2
11q22.3	ATM	Ataxia telangiectasia mutated
11q23-q24	LOH11CR2A; BCSC1	Loss of heterozygosity, 11, chromosomal region 2, gene A; breast cancer suppressor candidate 1
11q23.3	IGSF4; TSLC1; ST17; NECL2	Immunoglobin superfamily, member 4; tumor suppressor in lung cancer 1; suppression of tumorigenicity 17; nectin-like protein 2
12p13	CCND2	Cyclin D2
13q11-q12	LATS2	LATS, large tumor suppressor, homolog of 2 (Drosophila)
13q12.3	BRCA2; FANCD1	Breast cancer 2; Fanconi Anemia D1

Table 1. (Continued)

OMIM	Gene name(s)	Name of encoded protein(s)
13q14.1-q14.2	RB1	Retinoblastoma 1
13q14.3	ARL11; ARLTS1	ADP-ribosylation factor-like 11; ADP-ribosylation factor-like tumor suppressor 1
15q15.1	RAD51; RECA	RAD51, S. Cerevisiae, homolog of; recombination protein A
16p13.3	TSC2	Tuberous sclerosis 2; tuberin
16q12-q13	CYLD	Cylindromatosis
16q22.1	CTCF	CCCTC-binding factor (zinc finger protein)
16q22.1	CDH1	Cadherin 1
16q22.1	TERF2; TRF2	Telomeric repeat-binding factor-2
16q23.1	TERFIP	Telomeric repeat binding factor 2, interacting protein
16q22.1	FBXL8	F-box and leucine-rich repeat protein 8
16q22.1	LRRC29	Leucine rich repeat containing 29
16q22.3-q23.1	ATBF1	AT-binding transcription factor 1; alpha-fetoprotein enhancer binding protein
16q23.3-q24.1	WWOX	WW domain containing oxidoreductase
16q24.3	FBXO31	F-box protein 31
16q24.3	CBFA2T3 (B); MTG16	Core-binding factor, runt domain, alpha subunit 2; translocated to, 3; myeloid translocation gene on chromosome 16
16q24.3	CPNE7	Copine VII
16q24.3	CDK10; PISSLRE	Cyclin-dependent kinase 10
16q24.3	FANCA	Fanconi anemia, complementation group A
16q24.3	GAS11	Growth arrest specific 11
16q24.3	C16ORF3	Chromosome 16 open reading frame 3
17p11.2	MAP2K4; SERK1/SEK1; PRKMK4; MEK4	Mitogen-activated protein kinase kinase 4; SAPK/ERK kinase1; protein kinase, mitogen-activated, kinase 4; MAPK/ERK kinase 4
17p13.1	GABARAP	GABA(A) receptor-associated protein
17p13.1	TP53	Tumor protein 53
17p13.3	HIC1	Hypermethylated in cancer 1
17p13.3	OVCA1; DPH1; DPH2L1	Ovarian cancer-associated gene 1; DPH1 homolog (S. cerevisiae); diphtamidebiosynthesis protein 2, homolog-like 1 (S. cerevisiae)
17q21	BRCA1	Breast cancer 1
17q21.3	BECN1	Beclin 1 (coiled-coil, myosin-like BCL2 interacting protein)

OMIM	Gene name(s)	Name of encoded protein(s)
17q25.1	SLC9A3R1	Solute carrier family 9 (sodium/hydrogen exchanger), member 3 regulator 1
18p11.32	EPB41L3	Erythrocyte membrane protein band 4.1-like 3
18q21.1	SMAD4; ELAC1; DPC4	Mothers against DPP homolog 4 (Drosophila); elaC homolog 1 (E. coli); deleted in pancreatic cancer
18q21.3	DCC	Deleted in colorectal carcinoma; netrin-1 receptor
19p13.3	STK11; LKB1	Serine/threonine kinase 11
22q11	SMARCB1; BAF47; SNF	SWI/SNF related, matrix associated, actin dependent regulator of chromatin, subfamily b, member 1; Snf5, yeast, homolog of
22q12	RRP22	Ras-related on chromosome 22
22q12-q13	TMPRSS6	Transmembrane protease, serine 6 Matriptase 2
22q12.1	CHEK2; CHK2; RAD53	Checkpoint kinase 2, S.Pombe, homolog of
22q12.2	NF2	Neurofibromatosis type 2
22q13-q31	PRR5	Proline rich 5 (renal)

CLCA2 (1p31-p22)

It encodes a calcium-activated chloride channel. The 1p31 region is frequently deleted in sporadic breast cancer, suggesting that a TSG is present in this region. Absence of CLCA2 expression has been observed in several breast cancer tumors and cell lines, while it was found in normal breast epithelium. CLCA2 overexpression in CLCA2-negative cell lines (MDA-MB-231, MDA-MB-435) significantly reduced their tumorigenicity and metastasis capability. It appears that somatic mutations are not the major cause of CLCA2 gene silencing. On the other hand, CLCA2 is frequently inactivated in breast cancer by promoter region hypermethylation (epigenetic regulation), which makes it a candidate for the 1p31 breast cancer TSG (Gruber and Pauli 1999; Li *et al.* 2004a).

DIRAS3 (1p31)

It encodes a GTP-binding protein with 55-62% homology to Ras and Rap. In contrast to Ras, DIRAS3 inhibits growth, motility, and invasion. Reexpression of DIRAS3 in cancer cells inhibits signaling through Ras and PI3 kinase, upregulates $P21^{WAF1/CIP1}$, downregulates cyclin D1, induces JNK, and inhibits signaling through STAT3. Marked overexpression of DIRAS3 induces apoptosis. When DIRAS3 is expressed from a doxycycline-inducible promoter at more physiological levels, autophagy is induced, rather than apoptosis. Growth of breast cancer xenografts is reversibly suppressed by DIRAS3. DIRAS3 maps to a locus on human chromosome 1p31 that has been associated with a high frequency (40%) of LOH in breast and ovarian cancers. DIRAS3 is a maternally imprinted gene with methylation of the three CpG islands in the maternal allele of normal cells. It is expressed only from the paternal allele whose three CpG islands are not methylated. Loss of DIRAS3 expression is associated with tumor progression in breast cancer and decreased disease-free survival in ovarian cancer (Yu *et al.* 2005). This loss can occur through a genetic event, with LOH observed in 40% of breast, ovarian, and pancreatic cancers (Yu *et al.* 1999; Peng *et al.* 2000); but it can also occur through epigenetic mechanisms, and it has been suggested that acetylation and methylation of chromatin associated with the DIRAS3 promoter leads to loss of both DIRAS3 expression and the ability to suppress tumor growth. Changes in chromatin that silence DIRAS3 may be driven by methylation-dependent and -independent pathways. Reactivation of both the silenced paternal and imprinted maternal alleles can be achieved by demethylation and inhibition of histone deacetylation (Yu *et al.* 2003).

LPHH1 (1p31.1)

It encodes the human homologue of the rat latrophilin, a G-coupled, 7-span transmembrane protein that binds alpha-latrotoxin. It seems to be involved in the regulation of secretion (Bittner 2000). The effect of LPHH1 on breast cancer cell proliferation is unknown. Analysis of a panel of breast tumor cell lines revealed that a number apparently overexpressed LPHH1 whilst others showed very low levels of transcription. In one case, the overexpression correlated with a low level increase in gene copy number in the tumor line. No somatic LPHH1 mutations were detected through sequence analysis of four primary breast tumors that showed LOH at 1p31.1 (White *et al.* 2000). Additional data are needed to evaluate the potential role of LPHH1 as TSG.

TTC4 (1p31.3)

It encodes the fourth member of a family of genes containing a tetratricopeptide (TTC) repeat motif and a coiled-coil domain. This family has been implicated in a wide variety of functions, including tumorigenesis. The role of TTC4 in breast cancer cells is unknown. Examination of exon/intron structure of TTC4 and analysis of DNA from 20 sporadic breast tumors revealed polymorphic variations but no mutations affecting the open reading frame of TTC4 (Su *et al.* 1999; Su *et al.* 2000). Additional data are needed to conclude about the potential role of TTC4 as TSG.

RAD54L (1p32)

It encodes a protein that has been shown to play a role in homologous recombination related repair of DNA double-strand breaks.

RAD54L maps to chromosome 1p32 in a region of frequent LOH in several tumors, including breast cancers. For instance, in a series of 127 breast carcinomas, LOH was found in the RAD54L region in 20% of tumors (Gonzalez *et al.* 1999). RAD54L examination in several breast tumors and breast tumor cell lines revealed no coding sequence mutations (Rasio *et al.* 1997; Bell *et al.* 1999). However, missense mutations at functional regions of RAD54 and the absence of the wild-type RAD54 expression resulting from aberrant splicing has also been described in primary cancers (Matsuda *et al.* 1999).

FABP3 (1p33-p31)

Fatty acid metabolism in mammalian cells depends on a flux of fatty acids, between the plasma membrane and mitochondria or peroxisomes for beta-oxidation, and between other cellular organelles for lipid synthesis. FABP3 encodes a fatty acid-binding protein that play a role as transport vehicles of these hydrophobic compounds throughout the cytoplasm.

FABP3 immunoreactivity has been detected in epithelial cells of human breast tissue, but not on ductal carcinoma cells on the same sections.

FABP3 has antiproliferative activity for breast cancer cells *in vitro*. When these cells were transfected with a FABP3 expression construct, they exhibited differentiated morphology, reduced proliferation rate, reduced clonogenicity in soft agar, and reduced tumorgenicity in nude mice relative to mock-transfected or untransfected controls (Huynh *et al.* 1995).

Alteration analysis in 30 sporadic breast tumors indicated that 10 of these tumors showed LOH in the 1p32-p35 region, with 5 tumors showing LOH in the subregion containing the FABP3 gene. No mutations I FABP3 were found in this analysis. Despite experimental evidence that FABP3 has tumor suppressor activity, these data suggest that mutations in the coding region are uncommon in human breast tumorigenesis (Phelan *et al.* 1996). Hypermethylation of the FABP3 gene occurs frequently in breast cancer cell lines. A distinct methylation pattern is associated with loss of transcription and is reversible by treatment with 5-aza-deoxycytidine. Primary breast tumors also exhibited FABP3 gene methylation. Hypermethylation was correlated with the absence of FABP3 mRNA in these tumors. Our results suggest that epimutation of the FABP3 gene leads to silencing, which, in turn, may initiate or contribute to progression of breast cancer (Huynh *et al.* 1996).

RUNX3 (1p36)

In breast cancers, LOH is commonly observed at 1p36-ptel (Chin *et al.* 2006). RUNX3 encodes a protein involved in TGF-ß-induced tumor suppressor pathway. Gastric epithelial cells of RUNX3-null mice are resistant to the growth-inhibiting and apoptosis-inducing activity of TGF-ß (Fukamachi and Ito 2004). In 2002, a large body of evidence was presented to support a tumor suppressor role for RUNX3 in gastric cancer (Li *et al.* 2002). RUNX3 is frequently underexpressed in breast cancer compared with normal breast epithelium and its behavior supports a role of TSG (Bae and Choi 2004). Loss of RUNX3 function in primary breast cancers has been attributed to mislocalized protein expression (sequestration in the cytoplasm) and promoter hypermethylation (Kim *et al.* 2004a; Lau *et al.* 2006), but not to point mutation.

PRDM2(1) (1p36)

1p36 is a region commonly deleted in more than a dozen different types of human cancers, including breast (Weith *et al.* 1996) .The PRDM2 gene produces two protein products of different length, PRDM2(1) and PRDM2(2). PRDM2(2) is generated by an internal promoter and lacks an NH2-terminal motif of PRDM2(1), the PR (PRDI-BF1 and RIZ) domain conserved in a subfamily of zinc finger genes that function as negative regulators of tumorigenesis. PRDM2(1) is a histone methyltransferase and methylates lysine 9 in histone H3. This activity has been mapped to the PR domain.

Expression of PRDM2(1) is commonly decreased or at undetectable levels in breast cancer tissues and cell lines,as well as in other tumor types. Remarkably, PRDM2(2) is normally expressed in all cases examined, suggesting that the abnormality observed for PRDM2(1) is specific. PRDM2(1) silencing is correlated with CpG island promoter DNA methylation (Du *et al.* 2001). PRDM2(1) missense inactivating mutations and frameshift mutations that truncate a PR-interacting domain have also been observed (Kim *et al.* 2003).

Forced PRDM2(1) expression in breast cancer cells causes cell cycle arrest in G2-M and/or apoptosis. These observations suggest an exclusive negative selection for PRDM2(1) but not PRDM2(2) in breast cancer and a role for PRDM2(1) in tumor suppression (He *et al.* 1998).

SFN (1p36.11)

SFN is a direct target of the P53 tumor suppressor protein and its product inhibits cell cycle progression. In breast cancer cells, the SFN has been shown to interact with cyclin-dependent kinases and to control the rate of entry into mitosis. Recently, a proteomic analysis revealed that SFN regulates additional cellular processes relevant to carcinogenesis, as migration and MAP-kinase signaling.

The expression of SFN is down-regulated by CpG methylation in several types of human cancer, among them prostate, lung, breast and several types of skin cancer. SFN seems to be a marker specific for myoepithelial cells, and its expression could be related to a specific "basal/myoepithelial" biology of breast tumors (Simpson *et al.* 2004, Lacroix *et al.* 2004a).

DUTT1 (3p12.3)

Homozygous deletions or LOH at human chromosome band 3p12 are consistent features of various malignancies, including breast (Maitra *et al.* 2001). This suggests the presence of a TSG at this location. Only one gene, DUTT1, has been cloned thus far from the overlapping region deleted at 3p12 in several lung and breast cancer cell lines (Sundaresan *et al.* 1998; Angeloni *et al.* 2006). DUTT1, the human ortholog of the fly gene ROBO1 (Roundabout 1), has homology with neural cell adhesion molecule (NCAM) proteins. Extensive analyses of DUTT1 in lung cancer have not revealed any mutations (Angeloni *et al.* 2006). However DUTT1 methylation has been observed in breast tumors and 80% of breast showing methylation had allelic losses at 3p12, hence obeying Knudson's two hit hypothesis about TSG (Dallol *et al.* 2002).

PTPG (3p14.2)

Encodes protein tyrosine phosphatase gamma, which has been implicated as a TSG in kidney and lung cancers (Wang *et al.* 2006a). There are no consistent data about the PTPG gene in breast cancer. However, it has been reported that PTPG was deleted in benign proliferative breast disease associated with familial breast cancer and cytogenetic rearrangements of chromosome band 3p14 (Panagopoulos *et al.* 1996).

FHIT (3p14.2)

Common chromosome fragile sites show susceptibility to DNA damage, leading to alterations that contribute to cancer development. The cloning and characterization of fragile sites have demonstrated that fragile sites are associated with genes that relate to tumorigenesis. FHIT (fragile site FRA3B, at 3p14.2) and WWOX (fragile site 16D, at 16q23.3) are the most sensitive common fragile genes in the human genome. Both are putative TSGs.

FHIT protein is known to hydrolyze diadenosine triphosphate (Ap(3)A), however this hydrolase activity is not required for FHIT-mediated oncosuppression. Indeed, the molecular mechanisms and the regulatory elements of FHIT oncosuppression are largely unknown (Campiglio *et al.* 2006).

Restoration of fragile histidine triad (FHIT) expression was shown to induce apoptosis and to suppress tumorigenicity in breast cancer cell lines (Sevignani *et al.* 2003).

In an analysis of 46 sporadic invasive ductal breast carcinomas, evidence has been provided that biallelic inactivation of FHIT by LOH and hypermethylation leads to the complete inactivation of FHIT gene in patients with breast cancer (Yang *et al.* 2002a).

LOH at FHIT is associated with estrogen- and progesterone-negative breast tumors, high S-phase fraction, reduced patient survival. A multivariate analysis showed that LOH at FHIT results in a 60% increased relative risk of dying (Ingvarsson *et al.* 2001). In a study of 452 breast carcinomas, three distinct levels of FHIT expression were observed: in 154 cases (34.1%) expression was unchanged as compared to normal level; in 78 (17.2%) no expression was found; in the remaining 220 cases (48.7%), expression was intermediate. Overall, two-thirds of the cases had abnormal levels of the protein. Absence of FHIT was significantly associated with a higher grade and absence of hormone receptors (Ginestier *et al.* 2003). Loss of FHIT expression has been observed in up to 72%

of breast cancers and has been associated with increased p53, a high proliferation index, and increased tumor size and grade, and more generally, with poor prognostic markers (Arun *et al.* 2005). Breast carcinomas with basal and myoepithelial differentiation (Lacroix *et al.* 2004a) were associated with absence of expression of steroid hormone receptors and FHIT proteins and positive expression of p53 and EGFR (Rakha *et al.* 2006).

Of note, coordinately reduced FHIT and WWOX expression has been observed in in-situ breast cancer, and it has been suggested that this may contribute to the high-grade DCIS-invasive tumor pathway (Guler *et al.* 2005). FHIT and WWOX are also inactivated coordinately in invasive breast carcinoma (Guler *et al.* 2004).

PB1 (3p21)

It encodes a subunit of the human SWI/SNF chromatin remodeling complex, which maps to 3p21, in a region where frequent allele loss has been detected in breast, lung and kidney cancers (Horikawa and Barrett 2002). In 30 non-small-cell and 26 small-cell lung cancer cell lines, most of which had 3p21 allele loss, PB1 mRNA and protein expression were evaluated. In all cases, PB1 was expressed and no abnormal size PB1 protein was detected. No amino-acid sequence coding mutations was found in five non-small-cell and five small-cell lung cancer cell lines (Sekine *et al.* 2005). Extensive PB1 genetic and epigenetic analysis in breast cancer has not been performed to date.

RASSF1(A) (3p21.3)

LOH studies in lung, breast, and kidney tumors identified several loci in chromosome 3p likely to harbor one or more TSGs, including 3p21.3. An important TSG was suspected to reside at 3p21.3 because instability of this region is the earliest and most frequently detected deficiency in lung cancer. Overlapping homozygous deletions in lung and breast tumor cell lines reduced the critical region in 3p21.3 to 120 kb and this region was found to be exceptionally gene rich. From this critical region, eight genes were identified, including RASSF1. However, despite extensive genetic analysis in lung and breast tumors, none of these candidate genes were frequently (>10%) mutated (Lerman and Minna 2000).

RASSF1 binds Ras in a GTP-dependent manner and may serve as the effector that mediates Ras apoptotic effects. Alternatively, it may sequester RAS proteins thereby regulating the availability of these proteins for signaling.

Examination of RASSF1 revealed that one isoform, RASSF1(A) was lost in most lung tumor cell lines. Overexpression of RASSF1(A) but not the RASSF1(C) isoform in non–small cell lung cancer A549 cells reduced colony formation efficiency and suppressed growth of tumor cells in nude mice in vitro and in vivo growth assays, respectively. Subsequently, hypermethylation of the RASSF1(A) promoter region CpG island was identified as the major cause for loss of expression in a variety of tumors, including lung and breast cancer. Indeed, RASSF1A is inactivated almost exclusively by promoter region hypermethylation in lung, breast, and kidney cancers (Dammann et al. 2000; Agathanggelou et al. 2001) and mutations, apart from infrequent germ-line missense substitutions, are rare.

Percentage of RASSF1(A) methylation in breast tumors have been estimated between 35% and 62% (Dammann et al. 2000; Dammann et al. 2001; Burbee et al. 2001). Thus, RASSF1(A) falls into the category of genes frequently inactivated by methylation rather than mutational events. Hypermethylation profiling of 151 primary breast tumors with association to known prognostic factors in breast cancer was performed and RASSF1(A) hypermethylation was significantly more common in estrogen receptor-positive tumors (Shinozaki et al. 2005).

RBM5 (3p21.3)

It encodes a nuclear RNA binding protein with the ability to modulate both apoptosis and the cell cycle, and retard tumor formation. How RBM5 functions to carry out these, potentially interrelated, biological activities is unknown.

RBM5 has several important characteristics of a tumor suppressor, including both potentiation of apoptosis and inhibition of the cell cycle (Mourtada-Maarabouni et al. 2004).

In MCF-7 breast cancer cells that have lost the RBM5-containing region 3p21.3 (Forozan et al. 2000), overexpression of exogenous RBM5 was shown to enhance TNF-alpha-mediated apoptosis, suggesting that RBM5 may play a role in regulating the susceptibility of breast cancer cells to drug-induced apoptosis (Rintala-Maki et al. 2004). When RBM5 cDNA was introduced into human breast cancer cells that had 3p21-22 deletions, both anchorage-dependent and anchorage-independent growth was reduced (Oh et al. 2002).

No mutation in the RBM5 gene has been found in lung cancer cell lines (Lerman and Minna, 2000). Breast cancer and cell lines have not been examined.

TUSC4 (3p21.3)

A candidate TSG that has been identified in a 120-kb critical tumor homozygous deletion region (found in lung and breast cancers) of human chromosome 3p21.3 (Lerman and Minna 2000; Senchenko *et al.* 2003; Senchenko *et al.* 2004).

TUSC4 protein might be involved in mismatch repair and signaling to cell cycle checkpoints that activate apoptotic pathway(s) (Li *et al.* 2004b). TUSC4 has growth inhibitory activity for renal cell carcinoma, small cell lung carcinoma, and non-small cell lung carcinoma cell lines both *in vitro* and *in vivo* in mice.

Mutations in experimental tumors and intragenic homozygous deletions have been found in renal cell carcinoma, small cell lung carcinoma, non-small cell lung carcinoma, and other cancer cell lines (cervical HeLa, prostate LNCaP, and oral squamous SCC15). Preliminary analysis of EST databases also revealed the occurrence of nonsense and missense mutations in clones obtained from lymphoma, neuroblastoma, retinoblastoma, uterine, colon, brain, and other tumors. All of these features are consistent with the conclusion that TUSC4 is a multiple TSG (Li *et al.* 2004b). Extensive TUSC4 analysis has not been performed in breast cancer.

TMEM158 (3p21.3)

TMEM158 was identified in a screen as specifically upregulated during Ras-induced senescence. It is located at a chromosomal region, 3p21.3, frequently lost in several tumors types.

TMEM158 has been proposed to participate in anti-tumor responses that resemble cellular senescence.

To analyze the role of TMEM158 as a putative TSG in human breast cancer, TMEM158 mRNA expression was analyzed in 60 tumors. Decreased expression of TMEM158 was observed in 23% of the cases and overexpressed TMEM158 was detected in 15% of the primary breast tumors. A high frequency of LOH (30%) affecting the TMEM158 region was found. Statistically significant correlations were found between decreased TMEM158 expression and negative progesterone receptors, as well as between overexpressing TMEM158 tumors and high histological grade (Silva *et al.* 2006).

To analyze the physiological function of TMEM158, mutant mice deficient for this gene were generated. TMEM158-null mice were viable, fertile, developed normally and did not display any obvious abnormalities. Of relevance, TMEM158-deficient mice had a normal lifespan and did not exhibit predisposition to spontaneous tumors or to tumors induced by chemical carcinogens. Finally, TMEM158-deficient embryonic fibroblasts were indistinguishable from wild-type cells regarding their proliferation properties, immortalization, senescence and oncogenic transformation. These findings do not support a role of TMEM158 in tumor suppression or in oncogene-induced senescence (Nieto *et al.* 2006).

SEMA3B (3p21.3)

SEMA3B is one of the genes that have been identified as candidate TSGs at 3p21.3 since its downregulation and hypermethylation at its promoter regions were frequently detected in lung cancer. The 3p21.3 region is also frequently deleted in breast cancer (Tomizawa *et al.* 2001; Senchenko *et al.* 2004).

It encodes a secreted member of the semaphorin family, important in axonal guidance. SEMA3B induces apoptosis in lung and breast cancer (Castro-Rivera *et al.* 2004)

DNA methyltransferase 1 (DNMT1) is required to maintain DNA methylation patterns in mammalian cells, and is thought to be the predominant maintenance methyltransferase gene. RNA interference-mediated knockdown of DNMT1 protein expression resulted in >80% reduction of promoter methylation in re-expression of SEMA3B in a lung cancer cell line.

There is no data indicating mutation or promoter hypermethylation of SEMA3B in breast cancer.

TGFBR2 (3p22)

LOH is frequently observed at 3p22 in breast cancers (Maitra *et al.* 2001; Yang *et al.* 2002b)

TGF-beta inhibits the growth of most breast tumor cell lines. However, resistance to growth inhibition by TGF-ß has been demonstrated in a wide variety of human epithelial cell lines (Koli *et al.* 1997). Two of the TGF-ß receptors that mediate the actions of members of the TGF-ß family are trans-membrane serine/threonine kinases. TGF-ß binds directly to TGFBR2, a constitutively active kinase, and is then recognized by TGFBR1, which is directly phosphorylated and activated by TGFBR2.

Overexpression of a dominant-negative mutant form of the TGFBR2 in mammary epithelium results in lobular-alveolar hyperplasia and formation of mammary tumors (Gorska et al. 2003). Inactivating mutations in TGFBR2 or other TGF-ß signaling pathway genes, such as SMADs, are quite rare in breast cancers (Takenoshita et al. 1998; Lucke et al. 2001). However, loss or down-regulated expression of TGFBR2 in breast cancers has been shown through immunohistochemistry, and this reduced expression correlates with a higher tumor grade (Gobbi et al. 2000) and is inversely correlated with estrogen receptor-positivity (Sterling et al. 2006). Furthermore, decreased expression of TGFBR2 may be an early event in human breast tumorigenesis because women with breast biopsies containing epithelial hyperplasia lacking atypia and a reduced level of TGFBR2 immunostaining cells had a 3.41-fold increased risk for developing invasive breast cancer compared with women with similar lesions having high levels of TGFBR2 immunostaining (Gobbi et al. 1999).

It has been reported that TGFBR2 silencing involves histone deacetylation, instead of DNA methylation (Osada et al. 2005).

APRG1 (3p22.2)

It encodes a protein implicated in cell membrane interactions. Whether APRG1 may be genetically (mutation) or epigenetically (methylation) altered is unknown. Analysis of APRG1 expression in a series of 120 breast tumor tissues and 33 normal tissues was performed. APRG1 mRNA levels were lower in malignant tissues. There was a statistically significant reduction in APRG1 in grade 3 tumors cf. grade 1. APRG1 expression was highly negatively correlated with progressive disease. Additional data are needed to conclude about APRG1 acting as a TSG (Leris et al. 2005).

RARB(2) (3p24)

Frequent LOH at chromosome 3p22-24 has been reported in breast cancers (Yang et al. 2002b).

The biological effects of retinoids are mediated by retinoic acid receptors (RARs). One of them, RARbeta, is encoded by RARB, which is itself a retinoid target gene. RARB generates at least four distinct transcripts: splice variants RARB(1) and RARB(3) from transcription at promoter P1, and RARB(2) and RARB(4) from the retinoic acid receptor element-containing P2 promoter. In the human, only RARB(2) and RARB(4) transcripts have been identified in normal adult cells. The RARB(2) and RARB(4) transcripts differ only in the content of their 5'-most exon, a result of alternative splicing.

A growing body of evidence supports the hypotheses that the RARB(2) gene is a TSG and that the chemopreventive effects of retinoids are due to induction of RARB(2). Breast cancer cell lines SK-BR-3, T-47D, ZR-75-1, and MCF7 exhibited expression of RARB(2) only after demethylation and treatment with all-*trans*-retinoic acid. The first exon expressed in the RARB(2) transcript was methylated in cell lines ZR-75-1 and SK-BR-3. In all cell lines studied, both methylated and unmethylated alleles could be found. This observation suggests that biallelic inactivation is required for RARB(2) suppression. Six breast cancer specimens showed methylation in the same region of the gene. No expression of RARB(2) was found in any grade III lesion. An inverse association between methylation and gene expression was found in all grade II lesions. The RARB(2) gene from non-neoplastic breast tissue was unmethylated and expressed (Sirchia *et al.* 2000; Widschwendter *et al.* 2000). Hypermethylation profiling of 151 primary breast tumors with association to known prognostic factors in breast cancer revealed that RARB(2) gene hypermethylation was significantly more common in ERBB2-positive tumors (Shinozaki *et al.* 2005).

VHL (3p26-p25)

Eighty-two tumor specimens were screened for LOH at the VHL region, and compared to the adjacent, histologically normal tissue. Furthermore, mutations within the three exons of VHL in the same panel of tumors were analyzed. No mutation was found in the specimens examined. 29.2% of cases exhibited LOH at 3p25-26. Clinical and pathological data were available for all examined tumors; however no significant correlations were encountered. These results strongly indicate against a critical involvement of the tumor suppressor VHL in breast carcinogenesis (Sourvinos *et al.* 2001).

ATR (3q22-q24)

Mutations in BRCA1, BRCA2, ATM, TP53, CHEK2 and PTEN account for only 20-30% of the familial aggregation of breast cancer, which suggests the involvement of additional susceptibility genes.

ATR encodes a member of the PIK-related family which plays, along with ATM, a central role in cell-cycle regulation. ATR is essential for the maintenance of genomic integrity. It functions both in parallel and cooperatively with ATM, but whereas ATM is primarily activated by DNA double-strand breaks induced by ionizing radiation, ATR has been shown to respond to a much broader range of DNA damage. ATR has been shown to phosphorylate several tumor suppressors like BRCA1 and P53. ATR appears as a good candidate breast cancer susceptibility gene.

The entire coding region of the ATR gene was screened for mutations in affected index cases from 126 Finnish families with breast and/or ovarian cancer, 75 of which were classified as high-risk and 51 as moderate-risk families. However, this analysis did not support a major role for ATR mutations in hereditary susceptibility to breast and ovarian cancer (Heikkinen *et al.* 2005). The complete sequence of all exons and flanking intronic sequences were analyzed in DNA samples from 54 individuals affected with breast cancer from non-BRCA1/2 high-risk French Canadian breast/ovarian families. However, no deleterious mutations were identified in the ATR gene (Durocher *et al.* 2006).

SLIT2 (4p15.2)

Around 63% of breast tumors show LOH at 4p15.1–15.3 (Shivapurkar *et al.*1999).

The SLIT family is one of four conserved families of axonal guidance cues that have prominent developmental effects. The other three families are the netrins, the semaphorins and the ephrins (Yu and Bargmann 2001). Evidence is growing for the involvement of these guidance cues and their receptors in carcinogenesis. See for instance SEMA3B (semaphorin 3B) and DCC (the netrin-1 receptor).

Overexpression of SLIT2 was shown to suppress >70% of colony growth in breast cancer cell lines (with either absent or low SLIT2 expression). Because SLIT2 is primarily a secreted protein, SLIT2-conditioned medium suppressed the growth of several breast cancer lines (with absent or weak SLIT2 expression) by

26-51% but had no significant effect on a breast tumor cell line that expresses normal levels of SLIT2 (Dallol *et al.* 2002b).

SLIT2 is not commonly mutated in breast cancers. On the other hand, epigenetic inactivation of SLIT2 is frequently observed in these cancers. SLIT2 may be silenced by hypermethylation in breast cancer cell lines and is down-regulated in breast cancers in which it is methylated. For instance, SLIT2 promoter methylation has been detected in 59% of breast cancer cell lines. In these tumor lines, SLIT2 expression was restored by treatment with a demethylating agent. SLIT2 promoter methylation was detected in 43% of breast cancer. SLIT2 expression was down-regulated in methylated breast tumors, relative to normal control. The majority of methylated tumors demonstrated allelic loss at 4p15.2, which is consistent with Knudson's two-hit TSG hypothesis (Dallol *et al.* 2002b).

The putative SLIT2 receptor, DUTT1/ROBO1, is epigenetically inactivated in a subset of breast cancers. The finding of SLIT2 inactivation further strengthens the concept that ROBO1 loss or methylation will promote tumorigenesis.

In summary, SLIT2 appears as a convincing candidate for the breast TSG previously mapped to 4p15.2. SLIT2 resembles other TSGs such as RASSF1(A) in that epigenetic inactivation appears to be much more frequent than mutational mechanisms.

PRDM5 (4q26)

4q26 is a region thought to harbor TSG for several malignancies, including breast cancer.

PRDM5 encodes a protein that contains a PR domain. The gene has a CpG island promoter and is silenced in human breast, ovarian, and liver cancers. Overexpression of PRDM5 causes G_2/M arrest and apoptosis upon infection of tumor cells. These results suggest that inactivation of PRDM5 may play a role in carcinogenesis (Deng and Huang 2004).

HPGD (4q34-q35)

Prostaglandin E_2 (PGE$_2$) seems to have an important role in the development of breast cancer. High PGE$_2$ levels within breast tumors are associated with increased proliferation, invasiveness, resistance to apoptosis, and angiogenesis (Chang *et al.* 2004), and aberrant expression of cyclooxygenase-2 (COX-2), the rate-limiting enzyme in prostaglandin biosynthesis, can be found in the majority of breast cancers and is associated with an unfavorable outcome (Ristimaki *et al.* 2002). PGE_2 levels are regulated not only by its synthesis but also by its degradation. Encoded by HPGD, NAD^+-linked 15-hydroxyprostaglandin dehydrogenase is the key enzyme responsible for the biological inactivation of prostaglandins.

A tumor suppressor activity of HPGD has been identified in various cancers and epigenetic silencing of the enzyme by DNA methylation and histone modification has been suggested.

HPGD expression analysis in 8 breast cancer cell lines revealed low expression in all but one. In MDA-MB-231 cells, HPGD expression was up-regulated following demethylation treatment. Expression analysis of normal breast and breast cancer samples revealed low expression of HPGD in 16 (64%) of the tumors. In nine (36%) of the samples, the expression was <50% of control average. In a set of 28 breast cancer samples, higher HPGD mRNA expression was associated with ER expression and lower tumor stage, and borderline significance was noted for the association between low HPGD expression and lymphovascular invasion. Further analysis revealed methylation of the HPGD promoter in 30% of primary tumors. Transfection assays showed that transient up-regulation of HPGD levels in MDA-MB-231 cells resulted in a decreased clonal growth, and stable up-regulation significantly decreased the ability of these cells to form tumors in athymic mice. In contrast, transient silencing of HPGD in MCF-7 cells resulted in their enhanced proliferation, and a stable silencing in these cells enhanced cell cycle entry in vitro and tumorigenicity in vivo (Wolf *et al.* 2006).

It must be noted that loss of HPGD activity by LOH or mutation has not been described in colon, lung, bladder, or breast cancer.

DAB2 (5p13)

DAB2, also known as DOC2, has been previously proposed as a candidate TSG in ovarian cancers (Mok *et al.* 1998). It encodes a protein that negatively influences mitogenic signal transduction of growth factors and blocks Ras activity. DAB2 expression is lost in a majority of tumors, and homozygous deletions have been identified in a small percentage of tumors. DAB2 expression is absent or very low in a majority of breast and ovarian cancer cell lines. Transfection and expression of DAB2 in DAB2-negative MCF-7 and SK-Br-3 cells suppress tumorigenicity (He *et al.* 2001).

Frequent LOH at 5p13 has not been described in breast cancer. In contrast, 5p13 seems to be a site of recurrent high-level amplification (Forozan *et al.* 2000).

APC (5q21-q22)

This gene is mutant in familial adenomatous polyposis (FAP), an autosomal dominant disorder which typically presents with colorectal cancer. Its product is an important component of the Wnt signaling pathway (Polakis 1997), which binds to and inactivates ß-catenin.

There are few reports about the potential TSG role of APC in breast cancer. In a study of infiltrating lobular carcinomas, although no APC mutations were detected, promoter methylation (25/46, 52%) and LOH (7/30, 23%) of APC were found. Moreover, methylation of APC and CDH1 occurred concordantly (Sarrio *et al.* 2003). In a previous study of breast cancer patients, LOH affected loci in APC exons 11 and 15 in 9 of 35 (25%) and 4 of 34 (11%) heterozygous patients, respectively (Medeiros *et al.* 1994).

Despite the high rates of allelic loss in breast cancers, point mutations of the APC gene are infrequent in breast cancer. LOH at the APC locus and the methylation status of the APC gene promoter 1A were analyzed in 77 breast tumors and cell lines. LOH was observed in 63% of cases. The frequency of methylation in breast cancers increased with tumor stage and size (Virmani *et al.* 2001). Methylation and the lack of expression of APC were limited to the 1A promoter and its transcript. The consequences of APC gene promoter 1A methylation and the loss of expression of its specific transcript are not entirely clear. Breast and lung tumors frequently have weaker APC gene immunostaining than their adjacent nonmalignant epithelial cells. Loss of expression was observed in tumors irrespective of APC promoter 1A methylation, suggesting that additional mechanisms may be responsible for reduced expression of these genes in the various tumors studied. Methylation of a single promoter has been described for other genes having multiple promoters, including RARB(2) and RASSF1(A). In these genes, as with APC, methylation and loss of transcript expression are highly selective and always involve only a single specific promoter—the other promoter is never methylated. A significant trend between tumor size or stage and methylation frequency was noted in breast cancers. Both tumor size and stage are negative prognostic factors for breast cancer, suggesting that aberrant methylation of the APC promoter 1A is associated with breast cancer progression (Virmani *et al.* 2001).

IRF1 (5q31.1)

It encodes a transcription factor that is lost, mutated, or rearranged in renal and gastric cancers (Sugimura *et al.* 1997; Nozawa *et al.* 1998).

The IRF1 locus is 5q31.1; in 11% of sporadic breast cancers, 5q12–31 is deleted (Tirkkonen *et al.* 1998). However, no LOH or point mutation involving IRF1 has been described in breast tumors.

IRF1 is associated with growth suppression and apoptosis of breast cancer cells *in vitro* and decreases the tumorigenicity of cells inoculated into athymic nude mice. Loss of IRF1 activity, through the use of a dominant negative IRF1, enhances both the tumorigenicity and tumor growth rate of human breast cancer xenografts by affecting IRF1 dependent apoptosis and caspase activation (Kim *et al.* 2004b; Bouker *et al.* 2005).

PLAGL1 (6q24.2)

Loss of chromosome 6q21-qter is the second most frequent loss of chromosomal material in sporadic breast neoplasms suggesting the presence of at least one TSG on 6q.

Functional analysis of the protein encoded by PLAGL1 demonstrated that it may play a significant role as a transcription factor modulating growth suppression through mitogenic signaling pathways.

PLAGL1 is localized at chromosome 6q24-25, which is a frequent site for LOH in many solid tumors. It is in a chromosomal region maternally imprinted and linked to growth retardation in several organs and progression of disease states such as transient neonatal diabetes mellitus.

PLAGL1 expression is frequently down-regulated in breast carcinoma cells, although no mutation in PLAGL1 coding region was detected in a panel of 45 breast tumors with allelic imbalance of 6q24-q25 (Bilanges *et al.* 1999). In breast cancer, PLAGL1 is subject to two epigenetic processes, methylation of CpG islands and histone deacetylation, which may synergistically act to regulate the transcriptional silencing of the gene (Abdollahi *et al.* 2003).

LATS1 (6q24-q25.1)

Because LATS1-deficient mice develop soft tissue sarcomas or ovarian stromal cell tumors, LATS1 has been considered as a plausible TSG. In humans, LATS1 has been localized to chromosome 6q24-25.1. A frequent LOH at this locus has been reported in breast cancers (Fujii *et al.* 1996; Theile *et al.* 1996; Noviello *et al.* 1996).

Overexpression of LATS1 causes G_2-M arrest through the inhibition of CDC2 kinase activity in breast cancer cells *in vitro* and suppresses the tumorigenicity *in vivo* by inducing apoptosis (Takahashi *et al.* 2005).

No somatic mutation of LATS1 was reported in a study of 25 breast cancers (Morinaga *et al.* 2000). This suggests that loss of function of LATS1 is unlikely to be induced by the combination of somatic mutation and LOH but is more likely to be induced by other mechanisms such as hypermethylation.

In a series of 30 breast tumors, LATS1 promoter region was hypermethylated in 17 (56.7%) specimens. LATS1 level in breast tumors with hypermethylation was significantly lower than in those without hypermethylation. The decreased expression of LATS1 mRNA was significantly associated with a large tumor size, high lymph node metastasis, and estrogen receptor and progesterone receptor negativity. Furthermore, the decreased expression of LATS1 mRNA was significantly associated with a poor prognosis (Takahashi *et al.* 2005).

IGF2R (6q26)

It encodes the mannose 6-phosphate/insulin-like growth factor 2 receptor. IGF2R functions in the activation of TGFbeta, a potent growth inhibitor for most epithelial cells, the degradation of the mitogen, IGF2, and the intracellular trafficking of lysosomal enzymes (Da Costa *et al.* 2000).

LOH at the IGF2R locus on 6q26 has been demonstrated in approximately 30% of both invasive and in situ breast cancers. LOH was coupled with somatic point mutations in the remaining allele in several instances, leading to the proposition that IGF2R is a TSG (Hankins *et al.* 1996; Chappell *et al.* 1997; Oates *et al.* 1998). LOH at the IGF2R gene has been associated with poor differentiation at this early stage of breast cancer development and progression (Chappell *et al.* 1997).

ST7 (7q31.1-q31.2)

Many tumor types, including breast (Zenklusen *et al.* 1994), show high rates of LOH on chromosome 7q31. There is good evidence that ST7, which is located within the smallest common region of deletion at 7q31, is a major TSG at this locus (Zenklusen *et al.* 2001).

However, in a study of 149 primary ovarian, breast and colon carcinoma, no somatic mutation was found in ST7 (Thomas *et al.* 2001). Search for mutations in breast cancer cell lines revealed a complete wild-type sequence in all (Dong and Sidransky 2002; Brown *et al.* 2002). While ST7 promoter methylation has not been demonstrated, expression of the protein arginine methyltransferase 5 leads to reduced ST7 expression (Pal *et al.* 2004).

Functionally, ST7 behaves as a tumor suppressor in human cancer. ST7 suppressed growth of PC-3 prostate cancer cells inoculated subcutaneously into severe combined immunodeficient mice, and increased the latency of tumor detection from 13 days in control tumors to 23 days. Re-expression of ST7 was also associated with suppression of colony formation under anchorage-independent conditions in MDA-MB-231 breast cancer cells and ST7 mRNA expression was downregulated in 44% of primary breast cancers. Expression profiling of PC-3 cells revealed that ST7 predominantly induces changes in genes involved in re-modeling the extracellular matrix such as SPARC, IGFBP5 and several matrix metalloproteinases. These data suggest that ST7 may mediate tumor suppression mainly through modification of the tumor microenvironment (Hooi *et al.* 2006).

SFRP1 (8p12-p11.1)

It encodes a soluble Wnt antagonist and is located in a chromosomal region (8p22-p12) that is often deleted in breast cancer. The Wnt pathway is frequently altered in human cancers. In breast cancers, loss of SFRP1 expression in the absence of reduced gene copy number of SFRP1 has been observed (Armes *et al.* 2004).

SFRP1 expression has been inversely correlated with tumor stage and loss of SFRP1 expression in early stage breast tumors was associated with poor prognosis (Klopocki *et al.* 2004).

The role of epigenetic silencing of SFRP1 was examined in breast cancer cell lines and primary breast tumors. Methylation of SFRP1 was detected in 88% (7/8) of breast cancer cell lines, 17% (1/6) of grade 1 of ductal carcinoma in situ

(DCIS), 69% (9/13) of grade 2 and 3 of DCIS, 68% (19/28) of invasive ductal carcinomas (IDC) and 33% (6/18) of lobular carcinomas but not in any (0/14) of normal mammoplasty specimens and mammary epithelial organoids examined. Loss or downregulation of SFRP1 expression in tumors was frequently associated with promoter hypermethylation. In addition, breast cancer cell lines with SFRP1 promoter hypermethylation reexpressed SFRP1 mRNA after treatment with 5-azaC, implying that DNA methylation is the predominant epigenetic mechanism for SFRP1 gene silencing (Lo *et al.* 2006). In another study, mutation, methylation and expression analysis was performed in human primary breast tumours and breast cell lines. No SFRP1 gene mutations were detected. However, promoter methylation of SFRP1 was frequently observed in both primary breast cancer (61%, n=130) and cell lines. A tight correlation was found between methylation and loss of SFRP1 expression in primary breast cancer tissue. SFRP1 expression was restored after treatment of tumor cell lines with the demethylating agent 5-aza-2'-deoxycytidine (Veeck *et al.* 2006).

These findings suggest that frequent downregulation of SFRP1 expression in breast cancer can be attributed, in large part, to aberrant promoter hypermethylation in conjunction with or without histone deacetylation

DLC1 (8p21)

Frequent allelic loss is observed at 8p12-p22 in many neoplasms, including breast cancer. DLC1 is a candidate TSG in this region (Venter *et al.* 2005).

DLC1 encodes a Rho-GTPase–activating protein. Such proteins act as negative modulators of Rho proteins. The Rho proteins are members of the Ras superfamily and are involved in a variety of cellular functions, including the regulation of cell proliferation and actin cytoskeleton organization, and have been implicated in oncogenic transformation and cancer progression.

DLC1 study in various cancers has shown that it meets several criteria of a TSG. It is frequently inactivated due to genomic deletion or promoter hypermethylation in transformed cells, and its overexpression can result in the inhibition of in vitro colony formation, cell migration, and the suppression of tumor formation in immunocompromised mice.

DLC1 is often down-regulated or inactivated in breast primary tumors and breast tumor cell lines, and the restoration of its expression has been shown to significantly inhibit growth and tumorigenicity of cells derived from metastatic breast cancer (Yuan *et al.* 2003, Plaumann *et al.* 2003). Furthermore, DLC1 has recently been confirmed as a highly significant breast cancer susceptibility gene in a large-scale human genomic screening (Tang *et al.* 2004). In a clonal model of experimental organ-specific metastasis, DLC1 was found to be down-regulated in breast cell populations that were highly metastatic to bone (Kang *et al.* 2003). A role for DLC1 as tumor metastasis suppressor has also been shown (Goodison *et al.* 2005).

BNIP3L (8p21)

LOH at 8p12-p23 is one of the most frequent genetic events in breast cancer. BNIP3L encodes a protein that has sequence homology to pro-apoptotic proteins and is able to suppress colony formation in soft agar. However, BNIP3L expression was assessed in breast cancer cell lines and found to be expressed at similar levels relative to expression in their respective normal epithelial cell lines. Moreover, genetic analysis of BNIP3L in 25 primary breast tumors identified no mutation. These data suggest that BNIP3L is unlikely to be the target of 8p LOH in breast cancer (Lai *et al.* 2003).

RHOBTB2 (8p21.2)

Genomic deletions of the short arm of chromosome 8 are common in many human cancers and are frequently associated with a more aggressive tumor phenotype. One of the regions of LOH on 8p21-p22 contains two genes, LZTS1 (FEZ1) and RHOBTB2 (DBC2) that have been shown to be mutated at low frequency (Hamaguchi *et al.* 2002; Knowles *et al.* 2005).

Functional analysis revealed that RHOBTB2 expression in breast cancer cells lacking RHOBTB2 transcripts causes growth inhibition (Hamaguchi *et al.* 2002).

The biological roles of RHOBTB proteins remain unclear. To understand the physiological functions of RHOBTB2, a global approach was applied. Expression of RHOBTB2 was manipulated in HeLa cells and RNA profiling of the cells was performed by microarray analyses. Two networks were found to react substantially to RHOBTB2 expression; namely, more than half of participating genes are affected. One of the networks regulates cell growth through cell-cycle control and apoptosis. The other network is related to cytoskeleton and membrane trafficking. These findings suggest that the biological roles of RHOBTB2 are related directly and/or indirectly to these cellular machineries." (Siripurapu *et al.* 2005)

LZTS1 (8p22)

8p22 is a region frequently deleted in human tumors (Anbazhagan *et al.* 1998).

In gastric cancers, LZTS1 inactivation has been attributed to several factors including genomic deletion and methylation (Vecchione *et al.* 2001).

Alterations in LZTS1 expression have been observed in various cancers. LZTS1 expression was not detected in 15 of 15 breast cancer cell lines and 10 of 10 primary tumors (Ishii *et al.* 1999).

Introduction of LZTS1 into LZTS1-negative breast cancer cells resulted in suppression of tumorigenicity and reduced cell growth with accumulation of cells at late S-G$_2$/M stage of the cell cycle. LZTS1 is associated with microtubule components and interacts with CDC2 at late S-G$_2$/M stage in vivo. Thus, LZTS1 inhibits cancer cell growth through regulation of mitosis (Ishii *et al.* 2001).

MTUS1 (8p22)

MTUS1 encodes a family of proteins whose leader member, ATIP1, was previously isolated as an interacting partner of the angiotensin II (AT2) receptor involved in growth inhibition (Nouet *et al.* 2004). Alternative MTUS1 exon usage generates three major transcripts (ATIP1, ATIP3 and ATIP4), each showing different tissue distribution. ATIP polypeptides are identical in their carboxy-terminal region carrying four coiled-coil domains. In their amino-terminal portion, ATIP polypeptides exhibit distinct motifs for localization in the cytosol, nucleus or cell membrane, suggesting that MTUS1 gene products may be involved in a variety of intracellular functions in an AT2-dependent and independent manner. ATIP3 is the major transcript in tissues (prostate, bladder, breast, ovary, colon) corresponding to cancer types with frequent LOH at 8p22. High evolutionary conservation of ATIP amino-acid sequences suggests important biological roles for this new family of proteins in tumor suppression (Di Benedetto *et al.* 2006).

MCPH1 (8p23)

Deletion at 8p23 has been observed in breast tumors (Loo *et al.* 2004).

MCPH1, initially identified as an hTERT (telomerase) repressor, also functions as a proximal factor in the DNA damage checkpoints that control multiple damage sensors and early mediators. Disruption of MCPH1 function abolishes DNA damage responses and leads to genomic instability. Depletion of MCPH1 increased the accumulation of chromosomal aberrations.

Decreased levels of MCPH1 were detected in several types of human cancer, with MCPH1 expression being inversely correlated with genomic instability and metastasis. For instance, 72% of 54 breast cell lines tested showed decreases in MCPH1 DNA copy number. In comparing MCPH1 expression between nontransformed breast epithelial cells (HMEC, MCF10A, and MCF10F) and established breast cancer cell lines, significant decreases of MCPH1 RNA and protein expression were found in the breast cancer lines. MCPH1 expression was inversely correlated with the likelihood of breast cancer metastasis (van't Veer *et al.* 2002) and with the duration of relapse-free survival (Wang *et al.* 2005a).

Sequencing an entire 2.7 kb of MCPH1 cDNA from ten breast cancer specimens led to the identification of a 38 base pair MCPH1 deletion in exon 10 in one of the breast cancer specimens, which resulted in a premature stop codon in exon 11. These results suggest that MCPH1 functions as a TSG and that changes in MCPH1 levels could contribute to tumor progression through increasing genomic instability (Rai *et al.* 2006).

ST18 (8q11.2)

It encodes a zinc-finger DNA-binding protein that has the potential to act as transcriptional regulator. It lies within a frequently deleted region of chromosome 8q11.

ST18 is expressed in a number of normal tissues including mammary epithelial cells although the level of expression is quite low. In breast cancer cell lines and the majority of primary breast tumors, ST18 mRNA is significantly downregulated.

Ectopic ST18 expression in MCF-7 breast cancer cells strongly inhibits colony formation in soft agar and the formation of tumors in a xenograft mouse model.

A 160 bp region within the promoter of the ST18 gene is hypermethylated in about 80% of the breast cancer samples and in the majority of breast cancer cell lines. The strong correlation between ST18 promoter hypermethylation and loss of ST18 expression in tumor cells suggests that this epigenetic mechanism is responsible for tumor-specific downregulation (Jandrig *et al.* 2004).

CDKN2A (P14ARF) CDKN2A (P16INK4A) (9p21)

The CDKN2A locus encodes two (putative) tumor suppressor proteins, $P16^{INK4A}$ and $P14^{ARF}$, through use of alternative first exons. Both act in the two main cell-cycle control pathways, involving RB1 and P53 respectively. In fact, These proteins independently target two cell cycle control pathways, with $P16^{INK4A}$ inhibiting cyclin D1/cyclin-dependent kinases within the RB1 pathway and $P14^{ARF}$ inhibiting the oncoprotein MDM2 within the P53 pathway (Vestey *et al.* 2004)

The unusual genomic relationship of the open reading frames of these proteins initially fueled speculation that only one of the two was the true tumor suppressor, and loss of the other merely coincidental in cancer. Recent human and mouse genetic data, however, have firmly established that both proteins possess significant in vivo tumor suppressor activity, although there appear to be species- and cell-type specific differences between the two (Sharpless 2005).

Promoter hypermethylation of the $P16^{INK4A}$ and $P14^{ARF}$ genes is a major mechanism of their inactivation, followed by hemizygous deletions (Sharpless *et al.* 1999; Sherr and Weber 2000; Silva *et al.* 2003). Breast cancers rarely demonstrate homozygous deletions of either gene, with no mutations of $P14^{ARF}$ (Sharpless *et al.* 1999, Silva *et al.* 2003; Hui *et al.* 2000; Esteller *et al.* 2001).

SYK (9q22)

It encodes a protein-tyrosine kinase involved in coupling activated immunoreceptors to downstream signaling events that mediate diverse cellular responses, including proliferation, differentiation, and phagocytosis. SYK expression has been reported in cell lines of epithelial origin.

SYK is commonly expressed in normal human breast tissue, benign breast lesions, and low-tumorigenic breast cancer cell lines. SYK mRNA and protein, however, are low or undetectable in invasive breast carcinoma tissue and cell lines. Loss of SYK expression in breast tumors promotes tumor cell proliferation and invasion and predicts shorter survival of breast cancer patients (Coopman *et al.* 2000, Yuan *et al.* 2001).

Transfection of wildtype SYK into an SYK-negative breast cancer cell line markedly inhibited its tumor growth and metastasis formation in athymic mice. Conversely, overexpression of a kinase-deficient SYK in an SYK-positive breast cancer cell line significantly increased its tumor incidence and growth. Suppression of tumor growth by the reintroduction of SYK appeared to be the result of aberrant mitosis and cytokinesis. In addition to its well-known cytoplasmic localization, the full-length SYK is also present in the nucleus and that SYK nuclear translocation is a rate-limiting step to determine SYK tumor suppressor function. In fact, SYK acts as a transcription repressor in the cell nucleus, leading notably to the down-regulation of FRA1 and CCND1 oncogenes.

Thus, SYK is a potent modulator of epithelial cell growth and a potential tumor suppressor in human breast carcinomas (Coopman *et al.* 2000; Wang *et al.* 2005b).

Loss of SYK expression was associated to SYK promoter hypermethylation (Coopman *et al.* 2000, Yuan *et al.* 2001). Despite strong biological evidence, no mutations, translocation, or homozygous deletions involving the SYK gene have been reported in naturally occurring neoplasm.

DAB2IP (9q33.1-q33.3)

It encodes a member of the Ras GTPase-activating family. DAB2IP interacts directly with DAB2, also known as DOC2, which is a putative tumor suppressor in malignant cells, including mammary cancers. DAB2IP and DAB2 form a unique protein complex and have a negative regulatory activity to the Ras-mediated signal pathway (Wang *et al.* 2002).

Aberrant methylation is a major mechanism for down-regulation of DAB2IP gene and support the fact that the methylation-mediated transcriptional silencing of DAB2IP gene may be a critical event in tumorigenesis of breast cancer (Dote *et al.* 2004).

TSC1 (9q34) See TSC2, at 16p13.3 PTEN (10q23.3)

The protein encoded by the PTEN gene is a phosphatase. Though PTEN can dephosphorylate proteins, its primary biochemical and physiological targets are highly specialized plasma membrane lipids. These lipids, phosphatidylinositol-3,4,5-trisphosphate (PIP3) and phosphatidylinositol-3,4-bisphosphate are produced during cellular signaling events by the action of the lipid kinase phosphoinositide 3-kinase (PI3K). Thus, an elegant on-off switch has been evolved where the switch moves to "on" position when PI3K deposits a phosphate group on the D3 position of the inositol ring and is turned "off" when PTEN removes the phosphate group from the same position.

Cowden syndrome (CS) is a hamartoma syndrome. Affected members within CS kindred develop hamartomas of the hair follicle (trichilemmomas), the mucocutaneous membranes, breast, thyroid, and intestinal tissues. They are also at high risk for developing cancers of the breast and thyroid (Eng 2003).

Linkage analyses mapped the genetic locus for Cowden syndrome to the 10q23 region. This led to the cloning of PTEN and the discovery of germline PTEN mutations in 80% of families with CS. Thus, as with other TSGs, inheritance of a germline PTEN mutation results in the initiation of a cancer susceptibility syndrome (Sansal and Sellers 2004).

Sporadic PTEN alterations are not frequent events in breast cancers. In a number of cancers the rate of hemizygous inactivation events (LOH) in the 10q23 region significantly exceeds the rate of mutation of the remaining PTEN allele. For instance, though germline *PTEN* mutations in CS predispose to breast cancers, only infrequent *PTEN* mutations (6% to 7%) have been detected in the corresponding sporadic breast carcinomas (Feilotter *et al.* 1999; Freihoff *et al.* 1999).

Studies in tumors where LOH is common, but second mutations in PTEN are rare, including breast cancers have demonstrated loss of PTEN protein in 30% to 50% of samples (Depowski *et al.* 2001; Perren *et al.* 1999). In breast cancer this loss was strongly correlated with lymph node metastasis and with estrogen receptor–negative tumors (Perren *et al.* 1999). In another study, PTEN promoter hypermethylation was examined in 90 sporadic breast cancers, and its correlations with 11 molecular and pathologic parameters, including mRNA levels of PTEN was determined. The PTEN promoter was hypermethylated in 43 breast cancers (48%). PTEN hypermethylation was associated with ERBB2 overexpression, larger size, and higher histologic grade (Garcia *et al.* 2004).

PDCD4 (10q24)

PDCD4 expression is strongly induced during apoptosis in a number of cell types, and this seems achieved through interactions between PDCD4 and components of the translation initiation complex. Although PDCD4 has been proposed as a TSG (Goke *et al.* 2004; Palamarchuk *et al.* 2005), no LOH or point mutation involving this has been identified (Zhang *et al.* 2006).

MGMT (10q26)

DNA loss has been observed at 10q26-qter in breast cancer cell lines (Xie *et al.* 2002).

A number of DNA-damaging chemotherapeutic agents attack the O(6) position on guanine, forming the most potent cytotoxic DNA adducts known. The DNA repair enzyme O(6)-alkylguanine DNA alkyltransferase, encoded by the gene MGMT, repairs alkylation at this site and is responsible for protecting both tumor and normal cells from these agents. In breast cancer, MGMT also inhibits ER-mediated cell proliferation.

No LOH or point mutation involving MGMT has been described in breast cancer. In a series of 200 breast tumors, loss of MGMT expression was observed in 19% of cases. A significant correlation was seen between grade III tumor and loss of MGMT expression. Methylation-specific polymerase chain reaction in a subset of 20 cancers showed DNA methylation associated with the loss of MGMT expression (Munot *et al.* 2006).

WT1 (11p13)

In breast cancers, DNA loss is frequently observed at 11ptel-p15.5 (Chin *et al.* 2006). LOH involving WT1 was identified in 4/26 (15%) breast tumors (Fabre *et al.* 1999).

WT1 encodes a nuclear transcription factor that regulates the expression of the insulin-like growth factor (IGF) and transforming growth factor (TGF) systems, both of which are implicated in breast tumorigenesis.

Although originally identified as a TSG, WT1 is, however, overexpressed in a variety of hematologic malignancies and solid tumors, including breast cancer (Loeb and Sukumar 2002). Indeed, down-regulation of WT1 protein inhibits breast cancer proliferation (Zapata-Benavides *et al.* 2002). High expression of WT1 predicts poor prognosis in breast cancer patients (Miyoshi *et al.* 2002). WT1 protein was strongly expressed in primary carcinomas (27 of 31 tumors) but not in normal breast epithelium (1 of 20 samples). Additionally, the WT1 promoter was methylated in 6 of 19 (32%) primary tumors, which nevertheless expressed WT1. The promoter is not methylated in normal epithelium. Thus, although tumor-specific methylation of WT1 is established in primary breast cancer at a low frequency, other transcriptional regulatory mechanisms appear to supercede its effects in these tumors. These results suggest that WT1 might not have a tumor suppressor role in breast cancer (Loeb *et al.* 2001). There are, however, data consistent with a tumor suppressor role. For instance, MDA-MB-231-derived clones expressing WT1 in a stable manner exhibited reduced growth ability in soft agar and nude mice (Zhang *et al.* 2003).

The ability of WT1 to act as TSG could depend on p53 status of breast cancer cells (Idelman *et al.* 2003).

TSG101 (11p15.1-p15.2)

TSG101 was defined originally as a TSG, raising the expectation that absence of the encoded protein should lead to increased tumor cell growth and, perhaps, increased tumor cell aggressiveness. However, it was shown later that reduction of TSG101 protein has a negative impact on breast tumor cell growth, and that this gene is essential for the growth, proliferation, and survival of mammary epithelial cells (Wagner *et al.* 2003; Zhu *et al.* 2004).

CDKN1C (11p15.5)

Characterization of LOH at 11p15 in a panel of breast carcinomas demonstrated that DNA loss usually occurs at this locus. Analysis of the smallest region of overlap at this locus supported that the same gene or genes at 11p15 may be involved in Beckwith-Wiedemann syndrome (BWS), growth suppression detected by chromosome transfer, and breast cancer (Lichy *et al.* 1998). BWS is a congenital overgrowth condition with an increased risk of developing embryonic tumors, such as Wilms' tumor. A variety of molecular aberrations have been associated with BWS. The only mutations found within a gene at 11p15.5 are loss-of-function mutations in the CDKN1C gene, which codes for an imprinted cell-cycle regulator.

While point mutations have not been described in CDKN1C, aberrant methylation was detected in 11 of 18 (61%) and 17 of 38 (45%) breast cancer cell lines and tumors, respectively (Kobatake *et al.* 2004).

CST6 (11q13)

CST6 encodes a secreted inhibitor of lysosomal cysteine proteases capable of degrading extracellular matrix components.

CST6 is expressed in the normal human breast epithelium, but little or not at all in breast carcinomas and breast cancer cell lines. Ectopic expression of CST6 in human breast cancer cells suppresses cell proliferation, migration, invasion, and orthotopic tumor growth (Song *et al.* 2006).

CST6 hypermethylation has been observed in 12/20 (60%) primary breast tumors, indicating that this characteristic is common in breast malignancies (Ai *et al.* 2006). In a study of 12 breast cancer cell lines, seven (58%) lacked detectable expression of CST6 and treatment of these cells with 5-aza-2'-deoxycytidine resulted in a significant increase in CST6 expression, suggesting that the loss of expression may be related to methylation-dependent epigenetic silencing. In particular, hypermethylation of the proximal promoter was significantly associated with CST6 gene silencing, and methylation of a number of individual CpG was found to be statistically correlated with extinction of gene expression (Rivenbark *et al.* 2006).

IGSF4 (11q21-q24)

IGSF4 functions as a homophilic cell adhesion molecule.

LOH at the distal half of chromosome arm 11q is frequent in a variety of tumors, including breast cancer, and is often associated with poor prognosis. Thirty-one primary breast tumors showing LOH in 11q21-24 were analyzed for mutations in IGSF4. Intragenic alterations related to cancer were absent. The IGSF4 promoter region exhibited aberrant methylation patterns, and altogether 33% (10/30) of the successfully analyzed tumors showed evidence of elevated levels of IGSF4 CpG methylation. Ten percent (3/30) of the tumors showed significantly increased methylation. Thus, IGSF4 promoter region is frequently a second hit along with LOH in breast cancer (Allinen *et al.* 2002).

ATM (11q22.3)

ATM was originally identified by positional cloning as the gene that underlies the autosomal recessive condition ataxia-telangiectasia, which is a rare genomic instability syndrome.

It encodes a protein playing a central role in the complex processes that repair DNA DSB. ATM and CHEK2 are nuclear protein kinases that have been regarded as primary regulators of HR, the function of which is critical in determining which DSB repair mechanisms are recruited to initiate DSB repair. Both ATM and

CHEK2 interact physically with BRCA1, resulting in BRCA1 phosphorylation, leading to activation of its repair activity. It has been recently suggested that suggest that ATM and CHEK2, in addition of being HR regulatory proteins, act jointly to regulate the activity of BRCA1 in controlling the fidelity of DNA end-joining by precise NHEJ (Wang *et al.* 2006b).

Nearly 20 years ago, epidemiological surveys of relatives of ataxia-telangiectasia cases suggested that female relatives were at modestly increased risk of breast cancer. Subsequently, many studies have tried to clarify the role of ATM in breast cancer susceptibility, but have produced inconclusive and/or inconsistent results. Recently, large epidemiological and molecular studies have finally provided conclusive evidence that ATM mutations that cause ataxia-telangiectasia are breast cancer susceptibility alleles (Ahmed and Rahman 2006). Indeed, individuals from 443 familial breast cancer pedigrees and 521 controls were examined for ATM sequence variants and 12 mutations were identified in affected individuals and two in controls. The results demonstrate that ATM mutations that cause ataxia-telangiectasia in biallelic carriers are breast cancer susceptibility alleles in monoallelic carriers, with an estimated relative risk of 2.37. There was no evidence that other classes of ATM variant confer a risk of breast cancer (Renwick *et al.* 2006).

ATM is involved in the control of BRCA1 activity. BRCA1-mutant cancers are mostly, if not solely, "basal-like" tumors (Lacroix *et al.* 2004). In contrast, it seems that breast cancer occurring in carriers of ATM variants is not associated with distinctive histopathological features and does not resemble the tumor phenotype commonly observed in BRCA1 mutation carriers (Balleine *et al.* 2006).

LOH11CR2A (11q23-q24)

Frequent (ranging from 45–63%) allelic loss at human chromosome 11q23-q24 occurs in a wide variety of cancers, including breast cancer (Kerangueven *et al.* 1997; Laake *et al.* 1997), suggesting that this region may harbor a TSG. At least two independent regions of LOH at 11q23-q24 are present in breast cancer: the first region contains the ATM gene. A second, more telomeric region, is characterized by LOH frequencies at frequencies ranging from 40–60% in breast and various other cancers, suggesting that genes found within this region could reasonably be considered candidate TSG whose inactivation may be required in many of these tumors. LOH11CR2A (Monaco *et al.* 1997) has been identified in this region (Martin *et al.* 2003)

Northern analysis of the BCSC-1 mRNA revealed a lack of expression in 6 of 7 (86%) breast tumor cell lines, and its ectopic expression led to the suppression of colony formation in vitro and tumorigenicity in vivo (Martin *et al.* 2003)

RAD52 (12p13-p12.2)

In a series of 127 breast carcinomas, LOH was found in the RAD52 region in 16% of tumors (Gonzalez *et al.* 1999)

RAD52 was analyzed for the presence of germ-line mutations in 100 cases with early-onset breast cancer and for somatic mutations in 15 human breast cancer cell lines. Two premature stop codons, Ser346ter and Tyr415ter, were identified in germ-line RAD52 alleles from 5% of early-onset breast cancer cases. Together, these two heterozygous mutations were also found in 8% of a healthy control population, indicating that they do not confer an increased risk for breast cancer. RAD52 did not demonstrate somatic mutations in breast cancer cell lines. It is concluded that, despite its potential functional association with the BRCA gene products, RAD52 is not itself targeted by mutations in human breast cancer (Bell *et al.* 1999).

CCND2 (12p13.32)

The 12p13.32 region has not been described as frequently deleted by LOH in breast cancer. However, CCND2 expression is lost in most breast cancers. The frequency of cyclin D2 promoter hypermethylation in breast cancer and its absence in normal breast tissue and blood cells, as shown in this report, make it a candidate marker for breast malignancy (Evron *et al.* 2001).

LATS2 (13q11-q12)

LATS2 gene was mapped to chromosome 13q11-12. A frequent LOH of this locus has been reported in various cancers including breast (Emi *et al.* 1999). Overexpression of LATS2 causes G_1-S arrest through the inhibition of cyclin E/CDK2 *in vitro* as well as suppresses the tumorigenicity of NIH/v-ras–transformed cells *in vivo*, suggesting that LATS2 is a TSG (Takahashi *et al.* 2005).

Inactivation of a typical TSG is induced by mutation of one allele and LOH of the other allele, resulting in the complete loss of the gene function. With respect to LATS2, LOH is frequently observed in various human tumors, but only one mutation was reported in 60 esophageal tumors (breast cancer not studied) in the LATS2 gene (Ishizaki *et al.* 2002). These results seem to indicate that loss of function of LATS2 is unlikely to be induced by the combination of somatic mutation and LOH but is more likely to be induced by other mechanisms such as hypermethylation.

Methylation status of the promoter region of LATS2 as well as its correlation with its mRNA level was studied in human breast cancers. Correlation of LATS2 mRNA level with clinicopathologic characteristics of breast tumors was also studied. Of 30 breast tumors, LATS2 promoter region was hypermethylated in 15 (50.0%) specimens. LATS2 mRNA level in breast tumors with hypermethylation was significantly lower than those without hypermethylation. The decreased expression of LATS2 mRNA was significantly associated with a large tumor size, high lymph node metastasis, and estrogen receptor and progesterone receptor negativity. Hypermethylation of the promoter regions of LATS2 likely plays an important role in the down-regulation of its mRNA level in breast cancers, and breast cancers with a decreased expression of LATS2 mRNA level have a biologically aggressive phenotype (Takahashi *et al.* 2005).

RB1 (13q14.-q14.2)

RB1 plays a critical role in eukaryotic cell cycle progression, when cells exit G_0 or G_1 and enter S phase, thereby acting as a crucial negative regulator of cellular proliferation and neoplasia.

It has been shown that inactivation of RB1 and P53 in conjunction with the oncoproteins RAS and MYC and the telomerase subunit hTERT is sufficient to drive a number of normal human somatic cells to a tumorigenic fate (Kendall *et al.* 2005).

In 78 primary sporadic tumors, allelic imbalance was found in 30 cases (38%) (Hamann *et al.* 1996). In an analysis of genetic alterations in 47 primary breast tumors and 18 breast cancer cell lines, the most frequently lost TSG was RB1 (hemizygous loss in 26% of tumors) (Naylor *et al.* 2005).

ARL11 (13q14)

Deletions of regions at 13q14 have been detected by various genetic approaches in human cancers (Chen *et al.* 2001).

Encodes a member of ADP-ribosylation factor family.

The ARL11 Trp149Stop mutation has been shown to predispose to general familial cancer and high-risk familial breast cancer, provoking the attenuation of apoptotic function. In a study of 482 familial breast cancer cases (including 305 high-risk cases) and 530 control individuals, the ARL11 Cys148Arg variant revealed a significant association with an increased risk of high-risk familial breast cancer. On the basis of a small number of 46 cases, an association between the Trp149Stop mutation and an increased risk of bilateral BC was also shown (Frank *et al.* 2006).

In 4/7 breast cancer cell lines (57%), ARL11 was strongly down-regulated due to DNA methylation in its promoter region. After ARL11 restoration by adenoviral transduction, the homozygously ARL11-mutated MCF7 cells, but not cells expressing a normal ARL11 product, underwent apoptosis and inhibition of cell growth (Petrocca *et al.* 2006).

RAD51 (15q15.1)

Deficiencies in DNA repair can lead to carcinogenesis. Double-stranded DNA breaks (DSBs) may be the most detrimental form of DNA damage because, if left unrepaired, the detection of broken chromosomes will lead to cell death. Additionally, if DSBs are repaired improperly, they can result in chromosomal translocations and cancer. Central to the repair of DSBs by homologous recombination is RAD51, a homologue of the Escherichia coli DNA repair protein, RecA (Benson *et al.* 1994). RAD51 functions in DNA repair by mediating homologous pairing and strand exchange reactions.

RAD51 interacts (directly or indirectly) with a large number of proteins involved in DNA repair and the cell cycle. Interestingly, four of these proteins – BRCA1, BRCA2, TP53 and ATM – have been shown to be breast cancer predisposition genes in high-risk families. Alteration in either the expression or protein structure of RAD51 could therefore have similar deleterious effects on these essential pathways, leading to breast cancer.

Besides the interactions of RAD51 with key players in breast tumorigenesis, there is additional evidence to support a role for RAD51 in breast cancer. The RAD51 gene is located at chromosome position 15q15.1, a region shown to exhibit LOH in a large range of cancers, including those of the breast. In an analysis of 153 primary and metastatic carcinomas, 70% of cases exhibited a LOH (Wick *et al.* 1996). In a series of 127 sporadic breast carcinomas, LOH was found in the RAD51 region in 32% of tumors (Gonzalez *et al.* 1999).

There have been contrasting results about RAD51 expression in breast tumors. RAD51 mRNA expression in 16/16 of tumors from BRCA1/2 mutation-negative familial breast cancer patients was found to be one-half of that of the BT-474 breast cancer cell line (Hedenfalk *et al.* 2003), and protein levels were found to be decreased in 30% of breast tumors from a combination of sporadic and high-risk breast cancer patients (Yoshikawa *et al.* 2000). In contrast, there are reports of increased RAD51 expression in tumors and cancer cell lines. For instance, an increase in RAD51 mRNA expression in ductal carcinoma *in situ* (DCIS)-invasive ductal carcinoma (IDC) transition and high-tumor-grade breast cancers was found (Ma *et al.* 2003), while RAD51 overexpression was shown to correlate with histological grading of IDC (Maacke *et al.* 2000). There are numerous reports of RAD51 overexpression in a large range of cancer cell lines, including cervical cancer, prostate cancer and breast cancer (Raderschall *et al.* 2002).

In a screening of 93 early-onset (<40 years) breast cancer cases, 9% of which had a strong family history, for mutations in RAD51, a yeast-based protein truncation assay revealed no truncating mutations, and sequencing of a subset of 27 individuals with age at onset <30 years revealed no coding region variation. In the same study, a protein truncation assay of 15 breast cancer cell lines also revealed no truncating mutations (Bell *et al.* 1999).

In a screening of the RAD51 coding region and the surrounding intron/exon boundaries in 41 breast carcinomas (family history unknown), no mutation was found (Schmutte *et al.* 1999).

These RAD51 expression data are difficult to reconcile with a TSG function, as suggested by the LOH data.

TSC1 (9q34) TSC2 (16p13.3)

Tuberous sclerosis complex (TSC) is an autosomal dominant tumor syndrome that affects approximately 1 in 6000 individuals. It is characterized by the development of tumors, named hamartomas, in the kidneys, heart, skin and brain. The latter often cause seizures, mental retardation, and a variety of developmental disorders, including autism. This disease is caused by mutations within the tumor suppressor gene TSC1 (hamartin) on chromosome 9q34 or within TSC2 (tuberin) on chromosome 16p13.3. TSC patients carry a mutant TSC1 or TSC2 gene in each of their somatic cells, and LOH has been documented in a wide variety of TSC tumors. Recent data suggest that functional inactivation of TSC proteins might also be involved in the development of other diseases not associated with TSC, such as sporadic bladder cancer, breast cancer, ovarian carcinoma, gall bladder carcinoma, non-small-cell carcinoma of the lung, and Alzheimer's disease.

TSC1 and TSC2 form a heterodimer, suggesting they might affect the same processes. TSC2 is assumed to be the functional component of the complex and has been implicated in the regulation of different cellular functions. The TSC proteins regulate cell size control due to their involvement in the insulin signaling pathway. Furthermore, they are potent positive regulators of the cyclin-dependent kinase inhibitor p27, a major regulator of the mammalian cell cycle (Rosner *et al.* 2006)

Using immunohistochemical analysis, both TSC1 and TSC2 were found to be strongly stained in normal mammary epithelial cells and weakly in stromal cells. In invasive tumor tissues, however, the staining of both proteins was reduced. At mRNA level, although normal and tumor tissues expressed both TSC products, the transcript levels of TSC2 was significantly lower in tumor tissues compared with normal tissues. There was no statistical difference between node negative and node positive tumors with both TSC1 and TSC2. Tumors from patients who developed recurrence and died from breast cancer had significantly low levels of TSC2 compared with those who remained disease free. Likewise, TSC1 levels were significantly lower in patients with metastasis, recurrence and mortality, when compared with those remained disease free. Using methylation specific PCR, the TSC1 promoter was found to be heavily methylated in ZR751, MDA-MB-435, and BT549, but not in MCF-7 which expressed high level of TSC1. TSC1 promoter methylation was also seen in most breast tumors, but only in a limited number of normal tissues. The methylation of TSC2 promoter appears to be less frequent. MDA-MB-468, MDA-MB-483, MDA-MB-435S and weakly MDA-MB-435 were found to have methylated TSC2 promoter. In breast tissues, however, a very small number of samples were found to have methylation of the TSC2 promoter (Jiang *et al.* 2005).

CYLD (16q12–q13)

Cylindromas present most commonly as solitary and sporadic dermal nodules on the face and scalp. Cases of multiple cylindromas are dominantly inherited, and the neoplasms are referred to as "turban tumors" when multiple lesions cover the scalp. Primary cylindroma of the breast has been reported once in the past (Wang *et al.* 2004a).

CTCF (16q22)

CTCF is a widely expressed 11-zinc finger (ZF) transcription factor that is involved in different aspects of gene regulation including promoter activation or repression, hormone-responsive gene silencing, methylation-dependent chromatin insulation, and genomic imprinting.

CTCF has been proposed as a candidate TSG at 16q22.1. Enforced ectopic expression of CTCF inhibits cell growth in culture (Filippova *et al.* 1998).

No mutations were found in the CTCF gene in 125 samples of various tumors, including breast (Mironov *et al.* 1999). No mutations were found in a panel of tumor cell lines and primary tumors with and without loss of 16q (van Wezel *et al.* 2005).

A screening of more than 100 tumor samples for mutations that might disrupt CTCF activity did not reveal any CTCF mutations leading to truncations/premature stops. Rather, in breast, prostate, and Wilms' tumors, four different CTCF somatic missense mutations involving amino acids within the ZF domain were observed. Each ZF mutation abrogated CTCF binding to a subset of target sites within the promoters of certain genes involved in regulating cell proliferation but did not alter binding to the regulatory sequences of other genes. These observations suggest that CTCF may represent a novel tumor suppressor gene that displays tumor-specific "change of function" rather than complete "loss of function." (Filippova *et al.* 2002).

CDH1 (16q22.1)

It encodes a calcium dependent cell-cell adhesion glycoprotein involved in epithelial cell junctions.

Invasive lobular carcinoma (ILC) characteristically infiltrates diffusely as single cells. It has been shown that many of these tumors lack CDH1 expression. Indeed, most ILCs show genetic or epigenetic changes affecting CDH1 expression. For instance, in a study of 22 ILC, 12 samples (55%) were CDH1-negative. 17/22 (77%) of these tumors had methylation of the CDH1 promoter, including 11/12 (91%) of the CDH1-negative tumors. Five frameshift mutations, which resulted in downstream stop codons and one splice site mutation were identified in six different tumors (29%). 9/18 (50%) informative tumors showed LOH. In all cases in which there was loss of expression, this was consistent with biallelic inactivation of CDH1 by promoter methylation, mutation or allelic loss in any combination (Droufakou *et al.* 2001). Several different mechanisms (mutations, LOH, methylation) are involved in the frequent CDH1 inactivation in invasive, but also in *in situ* lobular breast cancer (Sarrio *et al.* 2003).

The frequency of LOH and the relationships between LOH and CDH1 loss of expression differ between ILC and invasive ductal carcinomas (IDC). For instance, 19% (18/97) of IDC showed complete loss of CDH1 protein expression compared with 64% (9/14) of ILC. LOH was detected in 46% (24/52) of IDC and 89% (8/9) of ILC. In the ILC, LOH was associated with complete loss of cell membrane expression of CDH1, although a cytoplasmic expression pattern was evident. In contrast, this association was not seen in the IDC (Ásgeirsson *et al.* 2000).

There are a limited number of studies directly correlating CDH1 methylation and CDH1 expression in the same sample of breast carcinomas. In one study, CDH1 promoter methylation was not uniformly associated with the loss of CDH1 expression. Overall, reduced expression of CDH1 (moderate, weak or absence of staining in cell membranes) was observed in 85% of our samples. Although not statistically significant, the intensity of CDH1 staining tended to diminish with methylation of the CDH1 promoter region: 65% of the IDCs (46 out of 71 cases) showed concomitant reduced levels of CDH1 and CDH1 hypermethylation. However, in 14 IDCs (20%), only unmethylated CDH1 alleles were detected despite reduced staining for CDH1. On the other hand, of the methylated tumors, 6 cases showed strong CDH1 staining. This indicates that additional mechanisms are involved in the loss or gain of CDH1 expression (LOH, gene mutation, changes in chromatin structure, and alterations of specific transcription pathways regulating the expression of the CDH1 gene (see for instance Peinado *et al.* 2004) (Caldeira *et al.* 2006).

Sporadic IDCs of the breast were tested for the 'two hits' required to inactivate CDH1. A high frequency (37.3%) of LOH was detected in 67 informative tumors, but no mutation was found. To examine the possibility that transcriptional mechanisms serve as the second hit in tumors with LOH, specific pathways, including genetic variant and hypermethylation at the promoter region and abnormal expression negative (Snail, see Liu *et al.* 2005) transcription factors, were identified. Of these, promoter hypermethylation and increased expression of Snail were found to be common (>35%), and to be strongly associated with reduced/negative CDH1 expression. However, unexpectedly, a significantly negative association was found between the existence of LOH and promoter hypermethylation, which contradicts the 'two-hit' model. Instead, since they coexisted in a high frequency of tumors, hypermethylation may work in concert with increased Snail to inactivate CDH1 expression. Given that CDH1 is involved in diverse mechanisms, loss of which is beneficial for tumors to invade but may also trigger apoptosis, this study suggests that maintaining a reversible mechanism, either by controlling the gene at the transcriptional level or by retaining an intact allele subsequent to LOH, might be important for CDH1 in IDC and may also be common in TSGs possessing diverse functions. These findings provide clues to explain why certain TSGs identified by LOH cannot fulfill the two-hit hypothesis (Cheng *et al.* 2001).

TERF2 (16q22.1), TERF2IP (16q23.1), FBXL8 (16q22.1) and LRRC29 (16q22.1) and FANCA (16q24.3)

Located in a region of frequent LOH, these genes were studied for insertion and deletion mutations and for expression differences in a panel of tumor cell lines and primary tumors with and without loss of 16q. None of the genes showed mutations or obvious expression differences. FANCA expression was shown to increase with tumor grade (van Wezel *et al.* 2005)

ATBF1 (16q22.3-q23.1)

The transcription factor ATBF1 at 16q22 was identified as a strong candidate TSG in prostate cancer, and loss of ATBF1 expression was associated with poorer prognosis in breast cancer.

Mutation, expression, and promoter methylation of ATBF1 were examined in 32 breast cancer cell lines. Only 2 of these cell lines had mutations, although 18 nucleotide polymorphisms were detected. In addition, 24 of 32 (75%) cancer cell lines had reduced ATBF1 mRNA levels, yet promoter methylation was not involved in gene silencing. These findings suggest that ATBF1 plays a role in breast cancer through transcriptional downregulation rather than mutations (Sun *et al.* 2006).

WWOX (16q23.1)

WWOX is a putative TSG involved in various tumors including breast cancer. High chromosomal abnormalities in a genomic region spanned by WWOX are associated with the fact that this gene covers approximately 1 million base pairs of the second most affected among common chromosomal fragile sites FRA16D.

Immunohistochemistry for cancer cells demonstrated that WWOX protein levels were not decreased but rather elevated in gastric and breast carcinoma, challenging the notion of WWOX as a classical TSG. In noncancerous cells, WWOX was observed only in epithelial cells, including mammary glands (Watanabe et al. 2003).

The relationship between WWOX mRNA levels, clinico-pathological factors, and other cancer related genes was evaluated in 132 cases of breast cancer. Expression of WWOX was higher in patients younger than 50 years old, in ER and PR positive tumors vs. negative for those receptors and tumors without lymph node metastasis vs. LN+. WWOX mRNA levels were also higher in tumors with higher apoptotic index (Bcl-2/Bax ratio). Negative associations were found between WWOX expression and cytokeratins 5/6 and 17, indicative of a basal-like phenotype of breast tumors. High level expression of WWOX was also associated with better disease free survival. Thus, reduced WWOX expression commonly observed in various neoplasias in cases of breast cancer is associated with markers of bad prognosis (Pluciennik et al. 2006).

Although, WWOX has been suggested as potential TSG, no inactivating mutations could be identified in this gene and it thus fail to fit the classic two-hit model for a TSG (van Wezel et al. 2005).

FBXO31 (16q24.3)

16q24.3 terminal band is one of the minimum regions of LOH (Cleton-Jansen et al. 2001). Among the genes present in this region, candidate TSGs were selected based on their known or predicted function as well as their expression in breast cancer cell lines (Powell et al. 2002). One candidate, FBXO31, was shown to induce cellular senescence in the breast cancer cell line MCF-7 and is probably the cellular senescence gene previously identified as SEN16 (Kaur et al. 2005).

FBXO31 has properties consistent with a tumor suppressor, because ectopic expression of FBXO31 in two breast cancer cell lines inhibited colony growth on plastic and inhibited cell proliferation in the MCF-7 cell line. Ectopic expression of FBXO31 in the breast cancer cell line MDA-MB-468 resulted in the accumulation of cells at the G_1 phase of the cell cycle. The expression of the FBXO31 gene was reduced in both breast tumor cell lines and sporadic primary breast tumors compared with nonmalignant breast epithelium. In addition, there was a significantly reduced expression in breast cancer cell lines with 16q LOH compared with those without 16q LOH. Similarly, in primary tumor samples, there was a trend for a higher proportion of tumors showing reduced expression when LOH of 16q was present. However, complete elimination of FBXO31 expression was not observed in breast tumors, because the maximum reduction of the relative FBXO31 expression was about 20% of the expression in normal breast. This suggests that down-regulation of FBXO31 is a likely scenario for function as a tumor suppressor but that residual levels of expression are retained (Kumar *et al.* 2005).

FBXO31 contains an F-box domain and is associated with the proteins Skp1, Roc-1, and Cullin-1, suggesting that FBXO31 is a component of a SCF ubiquitination complex. It has been proposed that FBXO31 may function as a tumor suppressor by generating SCF[(FBXO31)] complexes that target particular substrates, critical for the normal execution of the cell cycle, for ubiquitination and subsequent degradation (Kumar *et al.* 2005).

CBFA2T3 (B) (16q24.3)

The CBFA2T3-containing locus is frequently deleted in breast tumors. CBFA2T3 gene expression levels are aberrant in breast tumor cell lines and the B isoform CBFA2T3(B) is a potential TSG. No mutation has been identified in CBFA2T3 (van Wezel *et al.* 2005), but the gene is affected by aberrant promoter methylation and a statistically significant inverse correlation between aberrant CBFA2T3(B) promoter methylation and gene expression has been established (Bais *et al.* 2004).

CPNE7 (16q24.3)

Mutation analysis on 18 breast tumor tissue samples with ascertained LOH on chromosome 16q24.3 identified two polymorphisms, but no mutation in CPNE7. Information about CPNE7 methylation is not available as yet. Thus, there is no evidence to indicate that CPNE7 is a TSG at 16q24.3 involved in breast cancer (Savino *et al.* 1999).

FANCA (16q24.3)

FANCA mutation analysis of 19 breast tumors with specific LOH at 16q24.3 was performed. No tumor-specific mutation was found. Five polymorphisms were identified, but frequencies of occurrence did not deviate from those in a normal control population. Information about FANCA methylation is not available as yet. Thus, FANCA is likely not a TSG targeted by LOH at 16q24.3 in breast cancer (Cleton-Jansen *et al.* 1999).

CDK10 (16q24.3)

CDK10 encodes a putative cyclin-dependent kinase that, as with other members of this family, is likely to be involved in regulating the cell cycle and therefore may have a role in oncogenesis. Among the genes mapped to the frequently deleted 16q24.3 region, CDK10 was considered as a plausible candidate TSG. However, in breast tumors with ascertained LOH at 16q24.3, no variation was found in the coding sequence, suggesting that CDK10 is not a plausible TSG (Crawford *et al.* 1999)

GAS11 and C16orf3 (16q24.3)

GAS11 was identified in the smallest region of LOH common to breast and prostate at 16q24.3. It was viewed as a potential TSG due to the expression of its mouse homolog specifically during growth arrest. Another gene, C16orf3 (chromosome 16 open reading frame 3), was found to lie within intron 2 of GAS11. This apparently intronless gene is transcribed in the orientation opposite to that of GAS11, and is expressed at low levels. As these genes were not found to be mutated in breast tumor DNA, both were excluded as TSG (Whitmore *et al.* 1998).

MAP2K4 (17p11.2)

In breast cancers, DNA loss is frequently observed at 17p11.2-p12 (Chin *et al.* 2006). MAP2K4 encodes a member of the mitogen-activated protein kinases family of proteins, which function in signal transduction pathways that are involved in controlling key cellular processes, including apoptosis, in many organisms. In a set of 88 human cancer cell lines prescreened for LOH, two nonsense and three missense sequence variants of MAP2K4 were detected in cancer cell lines derived from human pancreatic, breast, colon, and testis cells. In vitro biochemical assays revealed that four of the five altered MAP2K4 proteins were inactive. These findings suggest that MAP2K4 may function as a TSG in certain types of cells (Teng *et al.* 1997).

MAP2K4 mutations or homozygous deletions have been reported in about 5-15% of breast cancer cells (Su *et al.* 1998; Su *et al.* 2002).

Recent data have suggested that MAP2K4 could function as a pro-oncogenic molecule instead of a suppressor in breast tumors. Indeed, ectopic expression of MAP2K4 by adenoviral delivery in MAP2K4-negative cancer lines stimulated the cell proliferation and invasion, whereas knockdown of MAP2K4 expression by small interference RNA in an MAP2K4-positive breast cancer cell line, MDA-MB-231, resulted in decreased anchorage-independent growth, suppressed tumor growth in mouse xenograft model, and increased cell susceptibility to apoptosis brought by stress signals such as serum deprivation (Wang *et al.* 2004b).

GABARAP (17p13.1)

There are at least seven commonly deleted regions on chromosome 17p13.1-p13.3 in sporadic breast cancer (Seitz *et al.* 2001). An attempt to identify new TSG in this region led to the identification of GABARAP.

Type-A receptors for the neurotransmitter GABA (gamma-aminobutyric acid) are ligand-gated chloride channels that mediate inhibitory neurotransmission. GABARAP encodes a protein associated to these receptors. GABARAP expression has, however, been found in many tissues, suggesting that it is also involved in biologic events other than interaction with GABA-A receptors (Wang *et al.* 1999).

GABARAP mRNA and protein expression are significantly down-regulated in breast tumors compared with normal tissue. Although neither gene mutation nor methylation of the promoter was found responsible for this decreased expression, 5-aza-2'-deoxycytidine (5-aza-dCyd) treatment was effective in gene up-regulation, suggesting a methylation-dependent upstream effect. Moreover, stable GABARAP transfectants were shown to have reduced growth rates and impaired colony-forming ability in soft agar in contrast to the control tumor cells. Furthermore, stable transfection resulted in suppression of tumorigenicity in nude mice. Thus, GABARAP is proposed to act as a putative TSG in breast cancer (Klebig *et al.* 2005).

HIC1 (17p13.3)

LOH at 17p is one of the most frequent genetic alterations in human cancers. Most often, allelic losses coincide with TP53 mutations at 17p13.1. However, in many types of solid tumors including sporadic breast cancers, frequent LOH or DNA methylation changes occur in a more telomeric region, at 17p13.3, in absence of any TP53 genetic alterations. Analyses of deletion mapping and CpG island methylation patterns have resulted in the identification of two candidate TSGs at 17p13.3, HIC1 and OVCA1.

HIC1 encodes a sequence-specific transcriptional repressor (Pinte *et al.* 2004). It is induced by p53 (Wales *et al.* 1995). HIC1 forms a transcriptional repression complex with SIRT1 deacetylase, and this complex directly binds the SIRT1 promoter and represses its transcription. Inactivation of HIC1 results in upregulated SIRT1 expression in normal or cancer cells; this deacetylates and inactivates p53, allowing cells to bypass apoptosis and survive DNA damage. Inhibition of SIRT1 function in cells without HIC1 abolishes the resistance to apoptosis (Chen *et al.* 2005).

In a study of 39 primary breast cancer tissues, virtually complete methylation of the HIC1 gene was found in 26 (67%) of the cases. LOH at the telomeric portion of chromosomal arm 17p was also found in 22 of the 26 cases with strongly methylated HIC1, suggesting that loss of an unmethylated HIC1 allele may contribute to the inactivation of HIC1 in cells with a pre-existing methylated allele. HIC1 was found to be expressed in microdissected normal breast ductal tissues and unmethylated tumors but not in tumors with hypermethylation of the HIC1 gene. These results indicate that hypermethylation of HIC1 and associated loss of HIC1 expression is common in primary breast cancer. Surprisingly, in all normal breast ductal tissues analyzed, approximately equal amounts of densely methylated HIC1 and completely unmethylated HIC1 were found. This is in contrast to most normal tissues, in which all copies of HIC1 are completely unmethylated. Thus, as the HIC1 gene is densely methylated in approximately one-half of the alleles in normal breast epithelium, this may predispose this tissue to inactivation of this gene by LOH (Fujii *et al.* 1998).

HIC1 promoter methylation, and allelic loss of a 700 kb region spanning the gene locus were analyzed in 33 invasive ductal carcinomas of the breast and 21 matched normal breast tissues. At least one genetic or epigenetic abnormality was found in 27 of the carcinomas tested (82%). Promoter methylation was demonstrated in 21 carcinomas (64%), and nine normal tissues (43%), whereas 18 malignant tumors (54%) showed allelic loss. Concomitant loss of heterozygosity and promoter hypermethylation in the region spanning HIC1 was detected in eight carcinomas (24%) suggesting that in this subset of tumors both copies of the gene are functionally lost (Parrella *et al.* 2005).

As no point mutations have been described in HIC1 (Chen and Baylin 2005), it seems that the gene is solely involved with epigenetic silencing in human cancer.

OVCA1 (17p13.3)

OVCA1 is a TSG identified by positional cloning from chromosome 17p13.3, a hot spot for chromosomal aberration in breast and ovarian cancers (Schultz *et al.* 1996).

OVCA1 is a component of the biosynthetic pathway of diphthamide on elongation factor 2, the target of bacterial ADP-ribosylating toxins (Nobukuni *et al.* 2005).

OVCA1 does not appear to be commonly mutated in breast tumors and related tumor cell lines. However, expression of OVCA1 is reduced in tumors. Exogenous expression of OVCA1 inhibited growth of ovarian cancer cells (Bruening *et al.* 1999).

OVCA1 acts as a tumor modifier in conjunction with TP53. Indeed, loss of one copy of OVCA1 can accelerate tumorigenesis and increase carcinoma incidence in a TP53+/- background. In addition, OVCA1 heterozygosity can modify tumor spectrum and increase multiple tumor burden in a TP53-/- background. Thus, the linkage of these tumor suppressor genes and their potential coordinated loss by chromosomal rearrangements may be an important mechanism for the phenotypic changes observed in tumors as they evolve (Chen and Behringer 2004).

BECN1 (17q21.3)

BECN1 is the first identified tumor suppressor protein that functions in the lysosomal degradation pathway of autophagy. In contrast to the ubiquitin-proteasome system which is the major cellular route for the degradation of short-lived proteins, autophagy is the major cellular route for the degradation of long-lived proteins and cytoplasmic organelles. Autophagy is a dynamic process involving the rearrangement of subcellular membranes to sequester cytoplasm and organelles for delivery to the lysosome where the sequestered cargo is degraded and recycled. BECN1 encodes a protein that interacts with the prototypic apoptosis inhibitor Bcl-2. Bcl-2 negatively regulates BECN1-dependent autophagy and BECN1-dependent autophagic cell death (Pattingre and Levine 2006).

BECN1 mapped to a tumor susceptibility locus, in a region approximately 150 kb centromeric to BRCA1, on chromosome 17q21 that is monoallelically deleted in 40% to 75% of cases of sporadic breast, ovarian, and prostate cancer (Aita *et al.* 1999).

BECN1 was shown to have tumor suppressor function in breast cancer cells; it reduced breast carcinoma cell proliferation, clonigenicity in soft agar, and tumorigenicity in nude mice (Liang *et al.* 1999).

Monoallelic BECN1 deletions have been identified in 9/22 (41%) breast cancer cell lines. Sequencing of genomic DNA from 10 of these cell lines revealed no mutations in coding regions or splice junctions. Additionally, Northern blot analysis of 11 cell lines did not identify any abnormalities in BECN1 transcripts (Aita *et al.* 1999). Although biallelic mutations of BECN1 have not yet been identified in human cancer, BECN1 is a haploinsufficient TSG in mice. Mice lacking one allele of BECN1 develop mammary neoplastic lesions and display an increased incidence of spontaneous malignancies, including B cell lymphomas, lung adenocarcinoma, and hepatocellular carcinoma (Qu *et al.* 2003; Yue *et al.* 2003).

SLC9A3R1 (17q25.1)

Frequent allelic loss is observed at 17q25.1 in primary breast cancers (Fukino *et al.* 1999).

SLC9A3R1 encodes a regulatory cofactor for epithelial Na+/H+ exchanger isoform 3, which interacts with ion transporters and receptors through its PDZ domains and with the MERM proteins (merlin, ezrin, radixin and moesin) via its carboxyl terminus. Thus, NHE-RF may act as a multifunctional adapter protein and play a role in the assembly of signal transduction complexes, linking ion channels and receptors to the actin cytoskeleton. SLC9A3R1 may also interact with the putative TSG SYK.

Intragenic mutation of SLC9A3R1 accompanied by LOH was found in approximately 3% (3/85) of breast cancer cell lines and primary breast tumors. Mutations occurred at the conserved PDZ domains at SLC9A3R1 NH2-terminus that bound to SYK, or at its COOH-terminus motif that binds to the product of NF2 putative TSG. SLC9A3R1 mutations decreased or abolished its interaction with SYK or NF2, suggesting a pathway link among these three molecules that may play a critical role in mammary neoplastic progression. Primary breast tumors with LOH at the SLC9A3R1 locus had clinical presentations of higher aggressiveness, indicating that deregulated SLC9A3R1 signaling might be associated with disease progression. Moreover, the LOH was inversely correlated with SYK promoter methylation, suggesting that SLC9A3R1 and SYK may transduce a common suppressive signal. Taken together, the results indicated SLC9A3R1 to be a candidate TSG in human breast carcinoma that may be interconnected to the SYK and NF2 suppressors." (Dai *et al.* 2004).

SLC9A3R1 is frequently expressed on luminal epithelial cells specialized in ion transport or absorption. Furthermore, estrogen receptor status and NHE-RF expression correlate closely in breast carcinoma specimens (Stemmer-Rachamimov *et al.* 2001).

EPB41L3 (18p11.32)

EPB41L3 localizes within chromosomal region 18p11.3, which is affected by LOH in various adult tumors, including breast cancer (Kittiniyom *et al.* 2001).

EPB41L3 encodes a member of the protein 4.1 superfamily, which encompasses structural proteins that play important roles in membrane processes via interactions with actin, spectrin, and the cytoplasmic domains of integral membrane proteins. Another member of the same family is the product of the NF2 gene, which has been proposed as TSG.

It seems that EPB41L3 functions as a growth suppressor by activating rac1-dependent c-Jun-NH2-kinase signaling (Gerber *et al.* 2006). Reintroduction of this protein into EPB41L3-null lung and breast tumor cell lines significantly reduced the number of cells, providing functional evidence that this protein possesses a growth suppressor function not confined to a single cell type.

From a study of 129 samples, it appears that, rather than point mutation, mechanisms such as imprinting or monoallelic expression in combination with LOH may be responsible for loss of the EPB41L3 protein in early breast disease." (Kittiniyom *et al.* 2004)

SMAD4 (18q21.1)

Transforming growth factor beta (TGF-beta) can act as suppressor and promoter of cancer progression in epithelial cells. Intracellular SMAD proteins play a pivotal role in mediating antimitogenic and proapoptotic effects of TGF-beta. SMAD4 inhibits tumor growth by inducing apoptosis in estrogen receptor-alpha-positive breast cancer cells (Li *et al.* 2005). More recently, a dual role has been observed for SMAD4, as it seems required for transforming growth factor beta-induced epithelial to mesenchymal transition and bone metastasis of breast cancer cells (Deckers *et al.* 2006).

SMAD4 expression is lower in human breast cancer than in surrounding breast epithelium (Stuelten *et al.* 2006).

SMAD4 is also known as "Deleted in Pancreatic Cancer 4 (DPC4), as both of its alleles are inactivated in nearly one-half of the pancreatic carcinomas.

SMAD4 is located on 18q21.1, a region frequently lost in breast cancers. However, point mutations of SMAD4 have been rarely observed. In an analysis of 338 tumors, originating from 12 distinct anatomic sites, sixty-four specimens were selected for the presence of the allelic loss of 18q and were further analyzed for SMAD4 sequence alterations. An alteration of the SMAD4 gene sequence was identified in one of eight breast carcinomas (Schutte *et al.* 1996). Two somatic biallelic lesions have been observed within and near SMAD4 in a breast cancer cell line (Jakob *et al.* 2005). More recently, homozygous SMAD4 deletions have been observed in two out of 24 primary infiltrative ductal carcinomas with 18q allelic imbalance (Zhong *et al.* 2006).

DCC (18q21.3)

DCC, as its name implies, has been shown to be frequently deleted in colorectal tumors. It encodes a receptor for netrin-1, known as axonal chemoattractant and survival factor.

It has been suggested that a TSG located at 18q21, but that is not SMAD4, might play a role in the development of some sporadic breast cancers, particularly those of the solid tubular type (Yokota *et al.* 1997).

LOH at the DCC locus was detected in 15 (51.7%) of 29 informative cases of primary breast cancers and 10 of 13 cases having DCC-LOH showed distinct reduction or loss of DCC expression (Kashiwaba *et al.* 1995).

In breast cancer LOH at 18q21.3 was found in 4 of 27 (15%) cases. In all cases of allelic loss the DCC locus or its proximal vicinity were involved. These alterations were only detected in large and undifferentiated tumors (Schenk *et al.* 1996).

STK11 (19p13.3)

In breast cancer, a high frequency of genomic deletion is found in chromosomal region 19p13. It has been suggested that 19p13.2-13.3 allele loss is a common event in the pathogenesis of breast carcinoma that often involves discontinuous LOH of multiple, localized TSGs (including STK11), the concurrent inactivation of which may contribute to breast cancer progression (Yang *et al.* 2004).

STK11 encodes a serine/threonine protein kinase. Germline mutations in STK11 are responsible for Peutz-Jeghers syndrome (PJS), a rare dominant disorder characterized by mucocutaneous pigmentation and gastrointestinal hematoma with an increased risk of developing cancer at multiple sites, including breast. Tumors associated with PJS have acquired somatic mutations in the remaining wild-type allele of STK11, strongly implicating STK11 as a tumor susceptibility gene (Ylikorkala *et al.* 1999). Most of the mutations in PJS families are point and truncation mutations within the kinase domain of STK11, suggesting that the kinase activity of STK11 is critical to its function.

Reintroduction of STK11 into breast cancer cell lines which lack the STK11 gene suppresses cell growth by G_1 cell cycle block. The STK11-mediated G_1 cell cycle arrest is caused by up-regulation of the expression of $P21^{WAF1/CIP1}$ in breast cancer cells (Shen *et al.* 2002).

A report of 31 sporadic breast cancers showed weak STK11 expression in 9 cases of cancer (Rowan *et al.* 2000). STK11 protein expression was evaluated in 116 breast cancers. It was correlated with higher histological grade, larger tumor size, presence of lymph node metastasis, and shorter survival (Shen *et al.* 2002). Among 70 invasive ductal carcinomas, loss of STK11 protein expression was recently shown to occur in a subset of high-grade carcinomas (Fenton *et al.* 2006).

SMARCB1 (22q11)

Organization of genomic DNA into chromatin aids in the regulation of gene expression by limiting access to transcriptional machinery. The SWI/SNF family of complexes, which are conserved from yeast to humans, are ATP-dependent chromatin-remodeling enzymes required for the transcription of a number of genes in yeast. In humans, the gene encoding the BAF47 subunit of the complex, located at 22q11.2, has been found to be mutated in a number of human tumors. In mice, loss of BAF47 results in highly penetrant cancer predisposition with 100%

of mice developing mature CD8(+) T cell lymphoma or rare rhabdoid tumors with a median onset of only 11 weeks (Roberts *et al.* 2002).

LOH has been reported for the BAF47 region in breast and liver cancer (Decristofaro *et al.* 2001). Whether BAF47 may act as a TSG in breast cancer remains, however, not documented.

RRP22 (22q12)

Ras proteins are members of a superfamily of related small GTPases. Some members are oncogenic, while other members seem to serve as tumor suppressors. Identified by using a bioinformatics approach, RRP22 inhibits cell growth and promotes caspase-independent cell death. Examination of neural tumor cells shows that RRP22 is frequently down-regulated due to promoter methylation. Moreover, reexpression of RRP22 in an RRP22-negative neural tumor cell line impairs its growth in soft agar. Unusually for a Ras-related protein, RRP22 localizes to the nucleolus in a GTP-dependent manner, suggesting a novel mechanism of action. Thus, RRP22 might serve as a potential tumor suppressor (Elam *et al.* 2005). To date, however, the role and status of RRP22 in breast cancer has not been documented.

TMPRSS6 (22q12-q13)

On chromosome 22q12-q13, several studies have reported allelic imbalance (AI) in different tumor tissues, including breast, and the region has been suggested as a possible location for a TSG (Allione *et al.* 1998; Iida *et al.* 1998; Castells *et al.* 2000; Hirano *et al.* 2001). By analysis of the 22q12-q13 region, TMPRSS6 was identified as associated to breast cancer risk (Hartikainen *et al.* 2006).

TMPRSS6 encodes a member of a family of type II transmembrane serine proteinases which have a possible role in cancer development. TMPRSS6 has the ability to degrade extracellular matrix components, suggesting that it may participate in some of the matrix-degrading processes occurring in both normal and pathologic conditions, including cancer progression. Because TMPRSS6 has only recently been discovered, little is known about its physiologic function(s). TMPRSS6 is expressed in normal breast tissue and the expression is elevated in breast cancer, which points out that TMPRSS6 is not expected to be a tumor suppressor.

CHEK2 (22q12.1)

CHEK2 encodes a protein that acts as an important signal transducer of cellular responses to DNA damage. It plays an important role in DSB responses leading to cell cycle checkpoint arrest, apoptosis, and DNA repair (see ATM for NHEJ). Activation of CHEK2 kinase in response to DNA damage is initiated by ATM-mediated phosphorylations. CHEK2 is a candidate TSG whose defects contribute to molecular pathogenesis of diverse types of human malignancies, both hereditary and sporadic.

The 1100delC, which abolishes the kinase function of CHEK2 (Wu *et al.* 2001), is a founder mutation, present in 5% of familial breast cancer cases without a mutation in the two known major breast cancer predisposition genes, BRCA1 and BRCA2 (Meijers-Heijboer *et al.* 2002). CHEK2 1100delC heterozygosity is associated with a three-fold risk of breast cancer in women in the general population (Weischer *et al.* 2006). Variants in CHEK2 other than 1100delC do not make a major contribution to breast cancer susceptibility (Schutte *et al.* 2003; Nevanlinna and Bartek 2006). The 1100delC mutation appears more prevalent among the patients with a positive ER status (4.2% vs. 1.0%) (de Bock *et al.* 2006).

Somatic mutations have been relatively rare in CHEK2, detected in various types of cancer, such as in some breast tumors (Ingvarsson *et al.* 2002; Sullivan *et al.* 2002)

Classically, the mechanism of tumorigenesis in association with tumor suppressor genes in inherited cancers involves the loss of the wt allele by LOH or by dominant-negative mode of action whereby the wt allele is prevented from carrying out its function by binding to the mutant allele. It has been shown that the mechanism of tumorigenesis in association with CHEK2 variants may not involve LOH (Sodha *et al.* 2002).

Methylation of CHEK2 has not been observed in breast carcinomas with downregulation of CHEK2 mRNA expression (Sullivan *et al.* 2002). In breast cancer, a very large number of tumor-specific splice variants have been detected, in addition to normal length mRNA, in all stage III breast tumors studied. It was suggested that extensive splicing variation of CHEK2 mRNA in breast tumors could be such a mechanisms, where splice variants may lack CHEK2 function or be mislocalized in cytoplasm (Staalesen *et al.* 2004).

NF2 (22q12.2)

Allelic losses on chromosome arm 22q are frequently observed in various carcinomas, including breast cancer.

NF2 encodes a protein named merlin, or schwannomin, which participate in a wide range of cell activities, in which the cytoskeleton latticework has important roles to play.

In order to examine the significance of NF2 in general carcinogenesis, comprehensive analysis of 68 cases of breast carcinoma, which shows frequent LOH at chromosome 22 was performed. No mutation was detected, suggesting that NF2 may be less important in the tumorigenesis of breast and liver cancers than in that of cancers originating from the neural crest (Kanai *et al.* 1995). NF2 gene aberrations were examined in another series of 60 breast tumors. A tumor-specific single-base substitution, resulting in an alteration of a single amino acid, was found in DNA from a breast cancer sample. This suggests possible but infrequent involvement of NF2 mutations in human breast cancers (Yaegashi *et al.* 1995). Somatic mutations of NF2 were screened in 55 breast cancers. No mutations were detected in any of the breast cancers (Arakawa *et al.* 1994).

PRR5 (22q13.31)

LOH at 22q13.31 is a frequent event during human breast carcinogenesis.

PRR5 encodes a proline-rich protein predominant in kidney. Mutational analysis of PRR5 in human breast tumors did not reveal somatic mutations. However, mRNA expression analyses revealed substantial downregulation of PRR5 expression in a subset of breast tumors and reduced expression in two breast cancer cell lines. Treatment with trichostatin A increased PRR5 mRNA levels in BT549 and MDA-MB-231 breast cancer cells, whereas 5'-aza-2'-deoxycytidine induced expression in MDA-MB-231 cells only. Thus, PRR5 may represent a potential candidate TSG in breast cancer (Johnstone *et al.* 2005).

Chapter 6

CONCLUSION

Many genes have been proposed as TSGs in breast cancer. While the implication of a few of them has been widely documented, much work is still in progress to establish the importance of others regarding their alteration frequency and even the extent of their participation to tumor formation.

Candidates TSGs are mostly related to DNA repair and recombination, apoptosis, cell survival, chromatin remodeling, Ras and/or Rho signaling pathways involved in growth, motility and invasion, TGF-beta suppressor pathway, P53 pathway.

The study of TSGs is complicated by the fact that they are often involved in overlapping pathways. Thus, various combinations of inactivation events may lead to different effects on cell behavior. This underlines the difficulty of developing successful TSG-targeted therapies.

ACKNOWLEDGMENTS

Many thanks to the "Fonds National de la Recherche Scientifique" (FNRS), the "Fonds de la Recherche Scientifique et Médicale" (FRSM), the "Biowin – Keymarker - Pôle Santé de Wallonie", the GIGA + PCRD + FP7 consortium, and also to Sophie Loubière. The author was partly supported by "Fondation Fornarina". This article is dedicated to the memory of Albert Lacroix (1935–2006). Merci pour toujours, Papa!

REFERENCES

Abdollahi, A; Pisarcik, D; Roberts, D; Weinstein, J; Cairns, P; Hamilton, TC. LOT1 (PLAGL1/ZAC1), the candidate tumor suppressor gene at chromosome 6q24-25, is epigenetically regulated in cancer. *Journal of Biological Chemistry*, 2003 278, 6041-6049.

Agathanggelou, A; Honorio, S; Macartney, DP; Martinez, A; Dallol, A; Rader, J; Fullwood, P; Chauhan, A; Walker, R; Shaw, JA; Hosoe, S; Lerman, MI; Minna, JD; Maher, ER; Latif, F. Methylation associated inactivation of RASSF1A from region 3p21.3 in lung, breast and ovarian tumours. *Oncogene*, 2001 20, 1509-1518.

Ahmed, M; Rahman, N. ATM and breast cancer susceptibility. *Oncogene*, 2006 25, 5906-5911.

Ai, L; Kim, WJ; Kim, TY; Fields, CR; Massoll, NA; Robertson, KD; Brown, KD. Epigenetic Silencing of the Tumor Suppressor Cystatin M Occurs during Breast Cancer Progression. *Cancer Research*, 2006 66, 7899-7909.

Aita, VM; Liang, XH; Murty, VV; Pincus, DL; Yu, W; Cayanis, E; Kalachikov, S; Gilliam, TC; Levine B. Cloning and genomic organization of beclin 1, a candidate tumor suppressor gene on chromosome 17q21. *Genomics*, 1999 59, 59-65.

Allinen, M; Peri, L; Kujala, S; Lahti-Domenici, J; Outila, K; Karppinen, SM; Launonen, V; Winqvist, R. Analysis of 11q21-24 loss of heterozygosity candidate target genes in breast cancer: indications of TSLC1 promoter hypermethylation. *Genes Chromosomes and Cancer*, 2002 34, 384-389.

Allione, F; Eisinger, F; Parc, P; Noguchi, T; Sobol, H; Birnbaum, D. Loss of heterozygosity at loci from chromosome arm 22Q in human sporadic breast carcinomas. *International Journal of Cancer*, 1998 75, 181-186.

Anbazhagan, R; Fujii, H; Gabrielson, E. Allelic loss of chromosomal arm 8p in breast cancer progression. *American Journal of Pathology*, 1998 152, 815-819.

Angeloni, D; ter Elst, A; Wei, MH; van der Veen, AY; Braga, EA; Klimov, EA; Timmer, T; Korobeinikova, L; Lerman, MI; Buys, CH. Analysis of a new homozygous deletion in the tumor suppressor region at 3p12.3 reveals two novel intronic noncoding RNA genes. *Genes Chromosomes and Cancer*, 2006 45, 676-691.

Arakawa, H; Hayashi, N; Nagase, H; Ogawa, M; Nakamura, Y. Alternative splicing of the NF2 gene and its mutation analysis of breast and colorectal cancers. *Human Molecular Genetics* 1994 3, 565-568.

Armes, JE; Hammet, F; de Silva, M; Ciciulla, J; Ramus, SJ; Soo, WK; Mahoney, A; Yarovaya, N; Henderson, MA; Gish, K; Hutchins, AM; Price, GR; Venter, DJ. Candidate tumor-suppressor genes on chromosome arm 8p in early-onset and high-grade breast cancers. *Oncogene*, 2004 23, 5697-5702.

Arun, B; Kilic, G; Yen, C; Foster, B; Yardley, DA; Gaynor, R; Ashfaq, R. Loss of FHIT expression in breast cancer is correlated with poor prognostic markers. *Cancer Epidemiology Biomarkers and Prevention*, 2005 14, 1681-1685.

Ásgeirsson, KS; Jónasson, JG; Tryggvadóttir, L; Ólafsdóttir, K; Sigurgeirsdóttir, JR; Ingvarsson, S; Ögmundsdóttir, HM. Altered expression of E-cadherin in breast cancer. patterns, mechanisms and clinical significance. *European Journal of Cancer*, 2000 36, 1098-1106.

Bae, SC; Choi, JK. Tumor suppressor activity of RUNX3. *Oncogene*, 2004 23, 4336-4340.

Bais, AJ; Gardner, AE; McKenzie, OL; Callen, DF; Sutherland, GR; Kremmidiotis G. Aberrant CBFA2T3B gene promoter methylation in breast tumors. *Molecular Cancer*, 2004 3, 2.2.

Balleine, RL; Murali, R; Bilous, AM; Farshid, G; Waring, P; Provan, P; Byth, K; Thorne, H; kConFab Investigators; Kirk, JA. Histopathological features of breast cancer in carriers of ATM gene variants. *Histopathology*, 2006 49, 523-532.

Bell, DW; Wahrer, DC; Kang, DH; MacMahon, MS; FitzGerald, MG; Ishioka, C; Isselbacher, KJ; Krainer, M; Haber, DA. Common nonsense mutations in RAD52. *Cancer Research*, 1999 59, 3883-3888.

Benson, FE; Stasiak, A; West, SC. Purification and characterization of the human Rad51 protein, an analogue of E. coli RecA. *EMBO Journal*, 1994 13, 5764-5771.

Bilanges, B; Varrault, A; Basyuk, E; Rodriguez, C; Mazumdar, A; Pantaloni, C; Bockaert, J; Theillet, C; Spengler, D; Journot, L. Loss of expression of the candidate tumor suppressor gene ZAC in breast cancer cell lines and primary tumors. *Oncogene*, 1999 18, 3979-3988.

Bittner, MA. Alpha-latrotoxin and its receptors CIRL (latrophilin) and neurexin 1 alpha mediate effects on secretion through multiple mechanisms. *Biochimie*, 2000 82, 447-452.

Borg, A. Molecular and pathological characterization of inherited breast cancer. *Seminars in Cancer Biology*, 2001 11, 375-385.

Bouker, KB; Skaar, TC; Riggins, RB; Harburger, DS; Fernandez, DR; Zwart, A; Wang, A; Clarke, R. Interferon regulatory factor-1 (IRF-1) exhibits tumor suppressor activities in breast cancer associated with caspase activation and induction of apoptosis. *Carcinogenesis*, 2005 26, 1527-1535.

Britschgi, C; Rizzi, M; Grob, TJ; Tschan, MP; Hugli, B; Reddy, VA; Andres, AC; Torbett, BE; Tobler, A; Fey, MF. Identification of the p53 family-responsive element in the promoter region of the tumor suppressor gene hypermethylated in cancer 1. *Oncogene*, 2006 25, 2030-2039.

Brown, VL; Proby, CM; Barnes, DM; Kelsell, DP. Lack of mutations within ST7 gene in tumour-derived cell lines and primary epithelial tumours. *British Journal of Cancer*, 2002 87, 208-211.

Bruening, W; Prowse, AH; Schultz, DC; Holgado-Madruga, M; Wong, A; Godwin, AK. Expression of OVCA1, a candidate tumor suppressor, is reduced in tumors and inhibits growth of ovarian cancer cells. *Cancer Research*, 1999 59, 4973-4983.

Burbee, DG; Forgacs, E; Zochbauer-Muller, S; Shivakumar, L; Fong, K; Gao, B; Randle, D; Kondo, M; Virmani, A; Bader, S; Sekido, Y; Latif, F; Milchgrub, S; Toyooka, S; Gazdar, AF; Lerman, MI; Zabarovsky, E; White, M; Minna, JD. Epigenetic inactivation of RASSF1A in lung and breast cancers and malignant phenotype suppression. *Journal of the National Cancer Institute*, 2001 93, 691-699.

Caldeira, JR; Prando, EC; Quevedo, FC; Neto, FA; Rainho, CA; Rogatto, SR. CDH1 promoter hypermethylation and E-cadherin protein expression in infiltrating breast cancer. *BMC Cancer*, 2006 6, 48.

Campiglio, M; Bianchi, F; Andriani, F; Sozzi, G; Tagliabue, E; Menard, S; Roz, L. Diadenosines as FHIT-ness instructors. *Journal of Cell Physiology*, 2006 208, 274-281.

Carter, RF. BRCA1, BRCA2 and breast cancer: a concise clinical review. *Clinical and Investigative Medicine*, 2001 24, 147-157.

Castells, A; Gusella, JF; Ramesh, V; Rustgi, AK. A region of deletion on chromosome 22q13 is common to human breast and colorectal cancers. *Cancer Research*, 2000 60, 2836-2839.

Castro-Rivera, E; Ran, S; Thorpe, P; Minna, JD. Semaphorin 3B (SEMA3B) induces apoptosis in lung and breast cancer, whereas VEGF165 antagonizes this effect. *Proceedings of the National Academy of Sciences of the United States of America*, 2004 101 11432-11437.

Chang, SH; Liu, CH; Conway, R; Han, DK; Nithipatikom, K; Trifan, OC; Lane, TF; Hla, T. Role of prostaglandin E2-dependent angiogenic switch in cyclooxygenase 2-induced breast cancer progression. *Proceedings of the National Academy of Sciences of the United States of America*, 2004 101, 591-596.

Chappell, SA; Walsh, T; Walker, RA; Shaw, JA. Loss of heterozygosity at chromosome 6q in preinvasive and early invasive breast carcinomas. *British Journal of Cancer*, 1997 75, 1324-1329.

Chen, C; Frierson, HF Jr; Haggerty, PF; Theodorescu, D; Gregory, CW; Dong, JT. An 800-kb region of deletion at 13q14 in human prostate and other carcinomas. *Genomics*, 2001 77, 135-144.

Chen, CM; Behringer, RR. Ovca1 regulates cell proliferation, embryonic development, and tumorigenesis. *Genes and Development*, 2004 18, 320-332.

Chen, WY; Wang, DH; Yen, RC; Luo, J; Gu, W; Baylin, SB. Tumor suppressor HIC1 directly regulates SIRT1 to modulate p53-dependent DNA-damage responses. *Cell*, 2005 123, 437-448.

Chen, WY; Baylin, SB. Inactivation of tumor suppressor genes: choice between genetic and epigenetic routes. *Cell Cycle*, 2005 4, 10-12.

Cheng, CW; Wu, PE; Yu, JC; Huang, CS; Yue, CT; Wu, CW; Shen, CY. Mechanisms of inactivation of E-cadherin in breast carcinoma: modification of the two-hit hypothesis of tumor suppressor gene. *Oncogene*, 2001 20, 3814-3823.

Chin, SF; Wang, Y; Thorne, NP; Teschendorff, AE; Pinder, SE; Vias, M; Naderi, A; Roberts, I; Barbosa-Morais, NL; Garcia, MJ; Iyer, NG; Kranjac, T; Robertson, JF; Aparicio, S; Tavare, S; Ellis, I; Brenton, JD; Caldas, C. Using array-comparative genomic hybridization to define molecular portraits of primary breast cancers. *Oncogene*, 2006 Sep 25; [Epub ahead of print].

Cleton-Jansen, AM; Moerland, EW; Pronk, JC; van Berkel, CG; Apostolou, S; Crawford, J; Savoia, A; Auerbach, AD; Mathew, CG; Callen, DF; Cornelisse, CJ. Mutation analysis of the Fanconi anaemia A gene in breast tumours with loss of heterozygosity at 16q24.3. *British Journal of Cancer*, 1999 79, 1049-1052.

Cleton-Jansen, AM; Callen, DF; Seshadri, R; Goldup, S; Mccallum, B; Crawford, J; Powell, JA; Settasatian, C; van Beerendonk, H; Moerland, EW; Smit, VT; Harris, WH; Millis, R; Morgan, NV; Barnes, D; Mathew, CG; Cornelisse, CJ. Loss of heterozygosity mapping at chromosome arm 16q in 712 breast tumors reveals factors that influence delineation of candidate regions. *Cancer Research*, 2001 61, 1171-1177.

Coopman, PJ; Do, MT; Barth, M; Bowden, ET; Hayes, AJ; Basyuk, E; Blancato, JK; Vezza, PR; McLeskey, SW; Mangeat, PH; Mueller, SC. The Syk tyrosine kinase suppresses malignant growth of human breast cancer cells. *Nature*, 2000, 406, 742-747.

Crawford, J; Ianzano, L; Savino, M; Whitmore, S; Cleton-Jansen, AM; Settasatian, C; d'apolito, M; Seshadri, R; Pronk, JC; Auerbach, AD; Verlander, PC; Mathew, CG; Tipping, AJ; Doggett, NA; Zelante, L; Callen, DF; Savoia A. The PISSLRE gene: structure, exon skipping, and exclusion as tumor suppressor in breast cancer. *Genomics*, 1999 56, 90-97.

Da Costa, SA ; Schumaker, LM ; Ellis, MJ. Mannose 6-phosphate/insulin-like growth factor 2 receptor, a bona fide tumor suppressor gene or just a promising candidate? *Journal of Mammary Gland Biology and Neoplasia*, 2000, 5 85-94.

Dai, JL; Wang, L; Sahin, AA; Broemeling, LD; Schutte, M; Pan, Y. NHERF (Na+/H+ exchanger regulatory factor) gene mutations in human breast cancer. *Oncogene*, 2004 23, 8681-8687.

Dallol, A; Da Silva, NF; Viacava, P; Minna, JD; Bieche, I; Maher, ER; Latif, F. SLIT2, a human homologue of the Drosophila Slit2 gene, has tumor suppressor activity and is frequently inactivated in lung and breast cancers. *Cancer Research*, 2002a 62, 5874-5880.

Dallol, A; Forgacs, E; Martinez, A; Sekido, Y; Walker, R; Kishida, T; Rabbitts, P; Maher, ER; Minna, JD; Latif F. Tumour specific promoter region methylation of the human homologue of the Drosophila Roundabout gene DUTT1 (ROBO1) in human cancers. *Oncogene*, 2002b 21, 3020-3028.

Dammann, R; Li, C; Yoon, JH; Chin, PL; Bates, S; Pfeifer, GP. Epigenetic inactivation of a RAS association domain family protein from the lung tumour suppressor locus 3p21.3. *Nature Genetics*, 2000 25, 315-319.

Dammann, R; Yang, G; Pfeifer, GP. Hypermethylation of the cpG island of Ras association domain family 1A (RASSF1A), a putative tumor suppressor gene from the 3p21.3 locus, occurs in a large percentage of human breast cancers. *Cancer Research*, 2001 61, 3105-3109.

de Bock, GH; Mourits, MJ; Schutte, M; Krol-Warmerdam, EM; Seynaeve, C; Blom, J; Brekelmans, CT; Meijers-Heijboer, H; van Asperen, CJ; Cornelisse, CJ; Devilee, P; Tollenaar, RA; Klijn, JG. Association between the CHEK2*1100delC germ line mutation and estrogen receptor status. *International Journal of Gynecological Cancer*, 2006 16 Suppl 2, 552-555.

Deckers, M; van Dinther, M; Buijs, J; Que, I; Lowik, C; van der Pluijm, G; ten Dijke, P. The tumor suppressor Smad4 is required for transforming growth factor beta-induced epithelial to mesenchymal transition and bone metastasis of breast cancer cells. *Cancer Research*, 2006 66, 2202-2209.

Decristofaro, MF; Betz, BL; Rorie, CJ; Reisman, DN; Wang, W; Weissman, BE. Characterization of SWI/SNF protein expression in human breast cancer cell lines and other malignancies. *Journal of Cell Physiology*, 2001 186, 136-145.

Deng, Q; Huang, S. PRDM5 is silenced in human cancers and has growth suppressive activities. *Oncogene,* 2004 23, 4903-4910.

Depowski, PL; Rosenthal, SI; Ross, JS. Loss of expression of the PTEN gene protein product is associated with poor outcome in breast cancer. *Modern Pathology*, 2001 14, 672-676.

Di Benedetto, M; Bieche, I; Deshayes, F; Vacher, S; Nouet, S; Collura, V; Seitz, I; Louis, S; Pineau, P; Amsellem-Ouazana, D; Couraud, PO; Strosberg, AD; Stoppa-Lyonnet, D; Lidereau, R; Nahmias, C. Structural organization and expression of human MTUS1, a candidate 8p22 tumor suppressor gene encoding a family of angiotensin II AT2 receptor-interacting proteins, ATIP. *Gene*, 2006 380, 127-136.

Dong, SM; Sidransky, D. Absence of ST7 gene alterations in human cancer. Clinical *Cancer Research*, 2002 8, 2939-2941.

Dote, H; Toyooka, S; Tsukuda, K; Yano, M; Ouchida, M; Doihara, H; Suzuki, M; Chen, H; Hsieh, JT; Gazdar, AF; Shimizu, N. Aberrant promoter methylation in human DAB2 interactive protein (hDAB2IP) gene in breast cancer. *Clinical Cancer Research*, 2004 10, 2082-2089.

Droufakou, S; Deshmane, V; Roylance, R; Hanby, A; Tomlinson, I; Hart, IR. Multiple ways of silencing E-cadherin gene expression in lobular carcinoma of the breast. *International Journal of Cancer*, 2001 92, 404-408.

Du, Y; Carling, T; Fang, W; Piao, Z; Sheu, JC; Huang, S. Hypermethylation in human cancers of the RIZ1 tumor suppressor gene, a member of a histone/protein methyltransferase superfamily. *Cancer Research*, 2001 61, 8094-8099.

Durocher, F; Labrie, Y; Soucy, P; Sinilnikova, O; Labuda, D; Bessette, P; Chiquette, J; Laframboise, R; Lepine, J; Lesperance, B; Ouellette, G; Pichette, R; Plante, M; Tavtigian, SV; Simard, J. Mutation analysis and characterization of ATR sequence variants in breast cancer cases from high-risk French Canadian breast/ovarian cancer families. *BMC Cancer* 2006 6, 230.

Elam, C; Hesson, L; Vos, MD; Eckfeld, K; Ellis, CA; Bell, A; Krex, D; Birrer, MJ; Latif, F; Clark GJ. RRP22 is a farnesylated, nucleolar, Ras-related protein with tumor suppressor potential. *Cancer Research*, 2005 65, 3117-3125.

Emi, M; Yoshimoto, M; Sato, T; Matsumoto, S; Utada, Y; Ito, I; Minobe, K; Iwase, T; Katagiri, T; Bando, K; Akiyama, F; Harada, Y; Fukino, K; Sakamoto, G; Matsushima, M; Iida, A; Tada, T; Saito, H; Miki, Y; Kasumi, F; Nakamura, Y. Allelic loss at 1p34, 13q12, 17p13.3, and 17q21.1 correlates with poor postoperative prognosis in breast cancer. *Genes Chromosomes and Cancer*, 1999 26, 134-141.

Eng, C. PTEN: one gene, many syndromes. *Human Mutation*, 2003 22, 183-198.

Esteller, M; Cordon-Cardo, C; Corn, PG; Meltzer, SJ; Pohar, KS; Watkins, DN; Capella, G; Peinado, MA; Matias-Guiu, X; Prat, J; Baylin, SB; Herman, JG. p14ARF silencing by promoter hypermethylation mediates abnormal intracellular localization of MDM2. *Cancer Research*, 2001 61, 2816-2821.

Esteller M. Dormant hypermethylated tumour suppressor genes: questions and answers. *Journal of Pathology*, 2005 205, 172-180.

Evron, E; Umbricht, CB; Korz, D; Raman, V; Loeb, DM; Niranjan, B; Buluwela, L; Weitzman, SA; Marks, J; Sukumar, S. Loss of cyclin D2 expression in the majority of breast cancers is associated with promoter hypermethylation. *Cancer Research*, 2001 61, 2782-2787.

Fabre, A; McCann, AH; O'Shea, D; Broderick, D; Keating, G; Tobin, B; Gorey, T; Dervan, PA. Loss of heterozygosity of the Wilms' tumor suppressor gene (WT1) in in situ and invasive breast carcinoma. *Human Pathology*, 1999 30, 661-665.

Feilotter, HE; Coulon, V; McVeigh, JL; Boag, AH; Dorion-Bonnet, F; Duboue, B; Latham, WC; Eng, C; Mulligan, LM; Longy, M. Analysis of the 10q23 chromosomal region and the PTEN gene in human sporadic breast carcinoma. *British Journal of Cancer*, 1999 79, 718-723.

Fenton, H; Carlile, B; Montgomery, EA; Carraway, H; Herman, J; Sahin, F; Su, GH; Argani, P. LKB1 protein expression in human breast cancer. *Applied Immunohistochemistry and Molecular Morphology*, 2006 14, 146-153.

Filippova, GN; Lindblom, A; Meincke, LJ; Klenova, EM; Neiman, PE; Collins, SJ; Doggett, NA; Lobanenkov, VV. A widely expressed transcription factor with multiple DNA sequence specificity, CTCF, is localized at chromosome segment 16q22.1 within one of the smallest regions of overlap for common deletions in breast and prostate cancers. *Genes Chromosomes and Cancer*, 1998 22, 26-36.

Filippova, GN; Qi, CF; Ulmer, JE; Moore, JM; Ward, MD; Hu, YJ; Loukinov, DI; Pugacheva, EM; Klenova, EM; Grundy, PE; Feinberg, AP; Cleton-Jansen, AM; Moerland, EW; Cornelisse, CJ; Suzuki, H; Komiya, A; Lindblom, A; Dorion-Bonnet, F; Neiman, PE; Morse, HC 3rd; Collins, SJ; Lobanenkov, VV. Tumor-associated zinc finger mutations in the CTCF transcription factor selectively alter tts DNA-binding specificity. *Cancer Research*, 2002 62, 48-52.

Forozan, F; Mahlamaki, EH; Monni, O; Chen, Y; Veldman, R; Jiang, Y; Gooden, GC; Ethier, SP; Kallioniemi, A; Kallioniemi, OP. Comparative genomic hybridization analysis of 38 breast cancer cell lines: a basis for interpreting complementary DNA microarray data. *Cancer Research*, 2000 60, 4519-4525.

Frank, B; Hemminki, K; Meindl, A; Wappenschmidt, B; Klaes, R; Schmutzler, RK; Untch, M; Bugert, P; Bartram, CR; Burwinkel B. Association of the ARLTS1 Cys148Arg variant with familial breast cancer risk. *International Journal of Cancer*, 2006 118, 2505-2508.

Freihoff, D; Kempe, A; Beste, B; Wappenschmidt, B; Kreyer, E; Hayashi, Y; Meindl, A; Krebs, D; Wiestler, OD; von Deimling, A; Schmutzler, RK. Exclusion of a major role for the PTEN tumour-suppressor gene in breast carcinomas. *British Journal of Cancer*, 1999 79, 754-758.

Fukamachi, H; Ito, K. Growth regulation of gastric epithelial cells by Runx3. *Oncogene*, 2004 23, 4330–4335.

Fukino, K; Iido, A; Teramoto, A; Sakamoto, G; Kasumi, F; Nakamura, Y; Emi, M. Frequent allelic loss at the TOC locus on 17q25.1 in primary breast cancers. *Genes Chromosomes and Cancer*, 1999 24, 345-350.

Fujii, H; Zhou, W; Gabrielson, E. Detection of frequent allelic loss of 6q23-q25.2 in microdissected human breast cancer tissues. *Genes Chromosomes and Cancer*, 1996 16, 35-39.

Fujii, H; Biel, MA; Zhou, W; Weitzman, SA; Baylin, SB; Gabrielson, E. Methylation of the HIC-1 candidate tumor suppressor gene in human breast cancer. *Oncogene*, 1998 16, 2159-2164.

Fukino, K; Iido, A; Teramoto, A; Sakamoto, G; Kasumi, F; Nakamura, Y; Emi, M. Frequent allelic loss at the TOC locus on 17q25.1 in primary breast cancers. *Genes Chromosomes and Cancer*, 1999 24, 345-350.

Garcia, JM; Silva, J; Pena, C; Garcia, V; Rodriguez, R; Cruz, MA; Cantos, B; Provencio, M; Espana, P; Bonilla, F. Promoter methylation of the PTEN gene is a common molecular change in breast cancer. *Genes Chromosomes and Cancer*, 2004 41, 117-124.

Gerber, MA; Bahr, SM; Gutmann, DH. Protein 4.1B/differentially expressed in adenocarcinoma of the lung-1 functions as a growth suppressor in meningioma cells by activating Rac1-dependent c-Jun-NH(2)-kinase signaling. *Cancer Research*, 2006 66, 5295-5303.

Ginestier, C; Bardou, VJ; Popovici, C; Charafe-Jauffret, E; Bertucci, F; Geneix, J; Adelaide, J; Chaffanet, M; Hassoun, J; Viens, P; Jacquemier, J; Birnbaum, D. Loss of FHIT protein expression is a marker of adverse evolution in good prognosis localized breast cancer. *International Journal of Cancer*, 2003 107, 854-862.

Gobbi, H; Simpson, JF; Borowsky, A; Jensen, RA; Page, DL. Metaplastic breast tumors with a dominant fibromatosis-like phenotype have a high risk of local recurrence. *Cancer*, 1999 85, 2170-2182.

Gobbi, H; Arteaga, CL; Jensen, RA; Simpson, JF; Dupont, WD; Olson, SJ; Schuyler, PA; Plummer, WD Jr; Page, DL. Loss of expression of transforming growth factor beta type II receptor correlates with high tumour grade in human breast in-situ and invasive carcinomas. *Histopathology*, 2000 36, 168-177.

Goke, R; Gregel, C; Goke, A; Arnold, R; Schmidt, H; Lankat-Buttgereit, B. Programmed cell death protein 4 (PDCD4) acts as a tumor suppressor in neuroendocrine tumor cells. *Annals of the New York Academy of Sciences*, 2004 1014, 220-221.

Gonzalez, R; Silva, JM; Dominguez, G; Garcia, JM; Martinez, G; Vargas, J; Provencio, M; Espana, P; Bonilla, F. Detection of loss of heterozygosity at RAD51, RAD52, RAD54 and BRCA1 and BRCA2 loci in breast cancer: pathological correlations. *British Journal of Cancer*, 1999 81, 503-509.

Goodison, S; Yuan, J; Sloan, D; Kim, R; Li, C; Popescu, NC; Urquidi V. The RhoGAP protein DLC-1 functions as a metastasis suppressor in breast cancer cells. *Cancer Research*, 2005 65, 6042-6053.

Gorska, AE; Shyr, YU; Aakre, M; Bhowmick, N; Moses, HL. Transgenic mice expressing a dominant-negative mutant type II transforming growth factor-ß receptor exhibit impaired mammary development and enhanced mammary tumor formation. *American Journal of Pathology*, 2003 163, 1539–1549.

Gruber, AD; Pauli, BU. Tumorigenicity of human breast cancer is associated with loss of the Ca2+-activated chloride channel CLCA2. *Cancer Research,* 1999 59, 5488-5491.

Guler, G; Uner, A; Guler, N; Han, SY; Iliopoulos, D; Hauck, WW; McCue, P; Huebner, K. The fragile genes FHIT and WWOX are inactivated coordinately in invasive breast carcinoma. *Cancer*, 2004 100, 1605-1614.

Guler, G; Uner, A; Guler, N; Han, SY; Iliopoulos, D; McCue, P; Huebner, K. Concordant loss of fragile gene expression early in breast cancer development. *Pathology International*, 2005 55, 471-478.

Hamaguchi, M; Meth, JL; von Klitzing, C; Wei, W; Esposito, D; Rodgers, L; Walsh, T; Welcsh, P; King, MC; Wigler, MH. DBC2, a candidate for a tumor suppressor gene involved in breast cancer. *Proceedings of the National Academy of Sciences of the United States of America*, 2002 99, 13647-13652.

Hamann, U; Herbold, C; Costa, S; Solomayer, EF; Kaufmann, M; Bastert, G; Ulmer, HU; Frenzel, H; Komitowski, D. Allelic imbalance on chromosome 13q: evidence for the involvement of BRCA2 and RB1 in sporadic breast cancer. *Cancer Research*, 1996 56, 1988-1990.

Hankins, GR; De Souza, AT; Bentley, RC; Patel, MR; Marks, JR; Iglehart, JD; Jirtle, RL. M6P/IGF2 receptor: a candidate breast tumor suppressor gene. *Oncogene*, 1996 12 2003-2009.

Hartikainen, JM; Tuhkanen, H; Kataja, V; Eskelinen, M; Uusitupa, M; Kosma, VM; Mannermaa, A. Refinement of the 22q12-q13 breast cancer--associated region: evidence of TMPRSS6 as a candidate gene in an eastern Finnish population. Clinical Cancer Research, 2006 12, 1454-1462.

He, L; Yu, JX; Liu, L; Buyse, IM; Wang, MS; Yang, QC; Nakagawara, A; Brodeur, GM; Shi, YE; Huang, S. RIZ1, but not the alternative RIZ2 product of the same gene, is underexpressed in breast cancer, and forced RIZ1 expression causes G2-M cell cycle arrest and/or apoptosis. *Cancer Research*, 1998 58, 4238-4244.

He, J; Smith, ER; Xu, XX. Disabled-2 exerts its tumor suppressor activity by uncoupling c-Fos expression and MAP kinase activation. *Journal of Biological Chemistry,* 2001 276, 26814-26818.

Hedenfalk, I; Ringner, M; Ben-Dor, A; Yakhini, Z; Chen, Y; Chebil, G; Ach, R; Loman, N; Olsson, H; Meltzer, P; Borg, A; Trent, J. Molecular classification of familial non-BRCA1/BRCA2 breast cancer. *Proceedings of the National Academy of Sciences of the United States of America*, 2003 100, 2532-2537.

Heikkinen, K; Mansikka, V; Karppinen, SM; Rapakko, K; Winqvist, R. Mutation analysis of the ATR gene in breast and ovarian cancer families. *Breast Cancer Research*, 2005 7, R495-R501.

Hirano, A; Emi, M; Tsuneizumi, M; Utada, Y; Yoshimoto, M; Kasumi, F; Akiyama, F; Sakamoto, G; Haga, S; Kajiwara, T; Nakamura, Y. Allelic losses of loci at 3p25.1, 8p22, 13q12, 17p13.3, and 22q13 correlate with postoperative recurrence in breast cancer. *Clinical Cancer Research*, 2001 7, 876-882.

Hohenstein, P; Giles RH. BRCA1: a scaffold for p53 response? *Trends in Genetics*, 2003 19, 489-494.

Hooi, CF; Blancher, C; Qiu, W; Revet, IM; Williams, LH; Ciavarella, ML; Anderson, RL; Thompson, EW; Connor, A; Phillips, WA; Campbell, IG. ST7-mediated suppression of tumorigenicity of prostate cancer cells is characterized by remodeling of the extracellular matrix. *Oncogene*, 2006 25, 3924-3933.

Horikawa, I; Barrett, JC. cDNA cloning of the human polybromo-1 gene on chromosome 3p21. *DNA Sequence*, 2002 13, 211-215.

Huang, J; Wei, W; Zhang, J; Liu, G; Bignell, GR; Stratton, MR; Futreal, PA; Wooster, R; Jones, KW; Shapero, MH. Whole genome DNA copy number changes identified by high density oligonucleotide arrays. *Human Genomics*, 2004 1, 287-299.

Hui, R; Macmillan, RD; Kenny, FS; Musgrove, EA; Blamey, RW; Nicholson, RI; Robertson, JF; Sutherland, RL. INK4a gene expression and methylation in primary breast cancer: overexpression of p16INK4a messenger RNA is a marker of poor prognosis. *Clinical Cancer Research*, 2000 6, 2777-2787.

Huynh, HT; Larsson, C; Narod, S; Pollak M. Tumor suppressor activity of the gene encoding mammary-derived growth inhibitor. *Cancer Research*, 1995 55, 2225-2231.

Huynh, H; Alpert, L; Pollak, M. Silencing of the mammary-derived growth inhibitor (MDGI) gene in breast neoplasms is associated with epigenetic changes. *Cancer Research*, 1996 56, 4865-4870.

Iau, PT; Macmillan, RD; Blamey, RW. Germ line mutations associated with breast cancer susceptibility. *European Journal of Cancer*, 2001 37, 300-321.

Idelman, G; Glaser, T; Roberts, CT Jr; Werner, H. WT1–p53 interactions in IGF-I receptor gene regulation. *Journal of Biological Chemistry*, 2003 278, 3474–3482.

Iida, A; Kurose, K; Isobe, R; Akiyama, F; Sakamoto, G; Yoshimoto, M; Kasumi, F; Nakamura, Y; Emi, M. Mapping of a new target region of allelic loss to a 2-cM interval at 22q13.1 in primary breast cancer. *Genes Chromosomes and Cancer*, 1998 21, 108-112.

Ingvarsson, S; Sigbjornsdottir, BI; Huiping, C; Jonasson, JG; Agnarsson, BA. Alterations of the FHIT gene in breast cancer: association with tumor progression and patient survival. *Cancer Detection and Prevention*, 2001 25, 292-298.

Ingvarsson, S; Sigbjornsdottir, BI; Huiping, C; Hafsteinsdottir, SH; Ragnarsson, G; Barkardottir, RB; Arason, A; Egilsson, V; Bergthorsson, JT. Mutation analysis of the CHK2 gene in breast carcinoma and other cancers. *Breast Cancer Research*, 2002 4, R4.

Ishii, H; Baffa, R; Numata, SI; Murakumo, Y; Rattan, S; Inoue, H; Mori, M; Fidanza, V; Alder, H; Croce, CM. The FEZ1 gene at chromosome 8p22 encodes a leucine-zipper protein, and its expression is altered in multiple human tumors. *Proceedings of the National Academy of Sciences of the United States of America*, 1999 96, 3928-3933.

Ishii, H; Vecchione, A; Murakumo, Y; Baldassarre, G; Numata, S; Trapasso, F; Alder, H; Baffa, R; Croce, CM. FEZ1/LZTS1 gene at 8p22 suppresses cancer cell growth and regulates mitosis. *Proceedings of the National Academy of Sciences of the United States of America*, 2001 98, 10374-10379.

Ishizaki, K; Fujimoto, J; Kumimoto, H; Nishimoto, Y; Shimada, Y; Shinoda, M; Yamamoto, T. Frequent polymorphic changes but rare tumor specific mutations of the LATS2 gene on 13q11-12 in esophageal squamous cell carcinoma. *International Journal of Oncology*, 2002 21, 1053-1057.

Jakob, J; Nagase, S; Gazdar, A; Chien, M; Morozova, I; Russo, JJ; Nandula, SV; Murty, VV; Li, CM; Tycko, B; Parsons, R. Two somatic biallelic lesions within and near SMAD4 in a human breast cancer cell line. *Genes Chromosomes and Cancer*, 2005 42, 372-383.

Jandrig, B; Seitz, S; Hinzmann, B; Arnold, W; Micheel, B; Koelble, K; Siebert, R; Schwartz, A; Ruecker, K; Schlag, PM; Scherneck, S; Rosenthal A. ST18 is a breast cancer tumor suppressor gene at human chromosome 8q11.2. *Oncogene*, 2004 23, 9295-9302.

Jiang, WG; Sampson, J; Martin, TA; Lee-Jones, L; Watkins, G; Douglas-Jones, A; Mokbel, K; Mansel, RE. Tuberin and hamartin are aberrantly expressed and linked to clinical outcome in human breast cancer: the role of promoter methylation of TSC genes. *European Journal of Cancer*, 2005 41, 1628-1636.

Johnstone, CN; Castellvi-Bel, S; Chang, LM; Sung, RK; Bowser, MJ; Pique, JM; Castells, A; Rustgi, AK. PRR5 encodes a conserved proline-rich protein predominant in kidney: analysis of genomic organization, expression, and mutation status in breast and colorectal carcinomas. *Genomics*, 2005 85, 338-351.

Kanai, Y; Tsuda, H; Oda, T; Sakamoto, M; Hirohashi, S. Analysis of the neurofibromatosis 2 gene in human breast and hepatocellular carcinomas. *Japanese Journal of Clinical Oncology*, 1995 25, 1-4.

Kang, Y; Siegel, PM; Shu, W; Drobnjak, M; Kakonen, SM; Cordon-Cardo, C; Guise, TA; Massague J. A multigenic program mediating breast cancer metastasis to bone. *Cancer Cell*, 2003 3, 537-549.

Karuman, P; Gozani, O; Odze, RD; Zhou, XC; Zhu, H; Shaw, R; Brien, TP; Bozzuto, CD; Ooi, D; Cantley, LC; Yuan, J. The Peutz-Jegher gene product LKB1 is a mediator of p53-dependent cell death. *Molecular Cell*, 2001 7, 1307-1319.

Kashiwaba, M; Tamura, G; Ishida, M. Frequent loss of heterozygosity at the deleted in colorectal carcinoma gene locus and its association with histologic phenotypes in breast carcinoma. *Virchows Archives*, 1995 426, 441-446.

Kaur, GP; Reddy, DE; Zimonjic, DB; de Riel, JK; Athwal, RS. Functional identification of a BAC clone from 16q24 carrying a senescence gene SEN16 for breast cancer cells. *Oncogene*, 2005 24, 47-54.

Kendall, SD; Linardic, CM; Adam, SJ; Counter, CM. A network of genetic events sufficient to convert normal human cells to a tumorigenic state. *Cancer Research*, 2005 65, 9824-9828.

Kerangueven, F; Noguchi, T; Coulier, F; Allione, F; Wargniez, V; Simony-Lafontaine, J; Longy, M; Jacquemier, J; Sobol, H; Eisinger, F; Birnbaum, D. Genome-wide search for loss of heterozygosity shows extensive genetic diversity of human breast carcinomas. *Cancer Research*, 1997 57, 5469-5474.

Kim, KC; Geng, L; Huang, S. Inactivation of a histone methyltransferase by mutations in human cancers. *Cancer Research*, 2003 63, 7619-7623.

Kim, TY; Lee, HJ; Hwang, KS; Lee, M; Kim, JW; Bang, YJ; Kang, GH. Methylation of RUNX3 in various types of human cancers and premalignant stages of gastric carcinoma. *Laboratory Investigations*, 2004a 84, 479-484.

Kim, PK; Armstrong, M; Liu, Y; Yan, P; Bucher, B; Zuckerbraun, BS; Gambotto, A; Billiar, TR; Yim, JH. IRF-1 expression induces apoptosis and inhibits tumor growth in mouse mammary cancer cells in vitro and in vivo. *Oncogene*, 2004b 23, 1125-1135.

Kittiniyom, K; Gorse, KM; Dalbegue, F; Lichy, JH; Taubenberger, JK; Newsham, IF. Allelic loss on chromosome band 18p11.3 occurs early and reveals heterogeneity in breast cancer progression. *Breast Cancer Research*, 2001 3, 192-198.

Kittiniyom, K; Mastronardi, M; Roemer, M; Wells, WA; Greenberg, ER; Titus-Ernstoff, L; Newsham IF. Allele-specific loss of heterozygosity at the DAL-1/4.1B (EPB41L3) tumor-suppressor gene locus in the absence of mutation. *Genes Chromosomes and Cancer*, 2004 40, 190-203.

Klebig, C; Seitz, S; Arnold, W; Deutschmann, N; Pacyna-Gengelbach, M; Scherneck, S; Petersen, I. Characterization of {gamma}-aminobutyric acid type A receptor-associated protein, a novel tumor suppressor, showing reduced expression in breast cancer. *Cancer Research*, 2005 65, 394-400.

Klopocki, E; Kristiansen, G; Wild, PJ; Klaman, I; Castanos-Velez, E; Singer, G; Stohr, R; Simon, R; Sauter, G; Leibiger, H; Essers, L; Weber, B; Hermann, K; Rosenthal, A; Hartmann, A; Dahl, E. Loss of SFRP1 is associated with breast cancer progression and poor prognosis in early stage tumors. *International Journal of Oncology*, 2004 25, 641-649.

Knowles, MA; Aveyard, JS; Taylor, CF; Harnden, P; Bass, S. Mutation analysis of the 8p candidate tumour suppressor genes DBC2 (RHOBTB2) and LZTS1 in bladder cancer. *Cancer Letters*, 2005 225, 121-130.

Knudson, AG Jr. Mutation and cancer: statistical study of retinoblastoma. *Proceedings of the National Academy of Sciences of the United States of America*, 1971 68, 820-823.

Kobatake, T; Yano, M; Toyooka, S; Tsukuda, K; Dote, H; Kikuchi, T; Toyota, M; Ouchida, M; Aoe, M; Date, H; Pass, HI; Doihara, H; Shimizu, N. Aberrant methylation of p57KIP2 gene in lung and breast cancers and malignant mesotheliomas. *Oncology Reports*, 2004 12, 1087-1092.

Koli, KM; Ramsey, TT; Ko, Y; Dugger, TC; Brattain, MG; Arteaga, CL. Blockade of transforming growth factor-ß signaling does not abrogate antiestrogen-induced growth inhibition of human breast carcinoma cells. *Journal of Biological Chemistry*, 1997 272, 8296-8302.

Kopelovich, L; Crowell, JA; Fay, JR. The epigenome as a target for cancer chemoprevention. *Journal of the National Cancer Institute*, 2003 95, 1747-1757.

Kumar, R; Neilsen, PM; Crawford, J; McKirdy, R; Lee, J; Powell, JA; Saif, Z; Martin, JM; Lombaerts, M; Cornelisse, CJ; Cleton-Jansen, AM; Callen, DF. FBXO31 is the chromosome 16q24.3 senescence gene, a candidate breast tumor suppressor, and a component of an SCF complex. *Cancer Research*, 2005 65, 11304-11313.

Kwabi-Addo, B; Giri, D; Schmidt, K; Podsypanina, K; Parsons, R; Greenberg, N; Ittmann, M. Haploinsufficiency of the Pten tumor suppressor gene promotes prostate cancer progression. *Proceedings of the National Academy of Sciences of the United States of America*, 2001 98, 11563–11568.

Laake, K; Odegard, A; Andersen, TI; Bukholm, IK; Karesen, R; Nesland, JM; Ottestad, L; Shiloh, Y; Borresen-Dale, AL. Loss of heterozygosity at 11q23.1 in breast carcinomas: indication for involvement of a gene distal and close to ATM. *Genes Chromosomes and Cancer*, 1997 18, 175-180.

Lacroix, M; Perec, G. A propos de données prétendument introuvables. *Bull Amat Belg Art Introuv*, 2003 1, 74-82.

Lacroix, M; Toillon, RA; Leclercq, G. Stable 'portrait' of breast tumors during progression: data from biology, pathology and genetics. *Endocrine-Related Cancer*, 2004a 11 497–522.

Lacroix, M; Leclercq, G. The 'portrait' of hereditary breast cancer. *Breast Cancer Research and Treatment*, 2005 89, 297–304.

Lacroix, M; Toillon, RA; Leclercq, G. p53 and breast cancer, an update. *Endocrine-Related Cancer*, 2006 13, 293-325.

Lacroix, M; Leclercq, G. 2006 Hereditary breast cancer: an update on genotype and phenotype. In New Breast Cancer Research, pp 27-51. Ed Andrew P. Yao. New York: Nova Science Publishers.

Lai, J; Flanagan, J; Phillips, WA; Chenevix-Trench, G; Arnold, J. Analysis of the candidate 8p21 tumour suppressor, BNIP3L, in breast and ovarian cancer. *British Journal of Cancer*, 2003 88, 270-276.

Lau, QC; Raja, E; Salto-Tellez, M; Liu, Q; Ito, K; Inoue, M; Putti, TC; Loh, M; Ko, TK; Huang, C; Bhalla, KN; Zhu, T; Ito, Y; Sukumar S. RUNX3 is frequently inactivated by dual mechanisms of protein mislocalization and promoter hypermethylation in breast cancer. *Cancer Research*, 2006 66, 6512-6520.

Leris, AC; Roberts, TR; Jiang, WG; Newbold, RF; Mokbel, K. Evidence for a tumour suppressive function of APRG1 in breast cancer. *Breast Cancer Research and Treatment*, 2005 93, 97-100.

Lerman, MI; Minna, JD. The 630-kb lung cancer homozygous deletion region on human chromosome 3p21.3: identification and evaluation of the resident candidate tumor suppressor genes. *Cancer Research*, 2000 60, 6116-6133.

Li, QL; Ito, K; Sakakura, C; Fukamachi, H; Inoue, K; Chi, XZ; Lee, KY; Nomura, S; Lee, CW; Han, SB; Kim, HM; Kim, WJ; Yamamoto, H; Yamashita, N; Yano, T; Ikeda, T; Itohara, S; Inazawa, J; Abe, T; Hagiwara, A; Yamagishi, H; Ooe, A; Kaneda, A; Sugimura, T; Ushijima, T; Bae, SC; Ito, Y. Causal relationship between the loss of RUNX3 expression and gastric cancer. *Cell*, 2002 109, 113–124.

Li, X; Cowell, JK; Sossey-Alaoui, K. CLCA2 tumour suppressor gene in 1p31 is epigenetically regulated in breast cancer. *Oncogene* 2004a 23, 1474-1480.

Li, J; Wang, F; Haraldson, K; Protopopov, A; Duh, FM; Geil, L; Kuzmin, I; Minna, JD; Stanbridge, E; Braga, E; Kashuba, VI; Klein, G; Lerman, MI; Zabarovsky, ER. Functional characterization of the candidate tumor suppressor gene NPRL2/G21 located in 3p21.3C. *Cancer Research*, 2004b 64, 6438-6443.

Li, Q; Wu, L; Oelschlager, DK; Wan, M; Stockard, CR; Grizzle, WE; Wang, N; Chen, H; Sun, Y; Cao, X. Smad4 inhibits tumor growth by inducing apoptosis in estrogen receptor-alpha-positive breast cancer cells. *Journal of Biological Chemistry*, 2005 280, 27022-27028.

Liang, XH; Jackson, S; Seaman, M; Brown, K; Kempkes, B; Hibshoosh, H; Levine, B. Induction of autophagy and inhibition of tumorigenesis by beclin 1. *Nature*, 1999 402, 672-676.

Lichy, JH; Zavar, M; Tsai, MM; O'Leary, TJ; Taubenberger JK. Loss of heterozygosity on chromosome 11p15 during histological progression in microdissected ductal carcinoma of the breast. *American Journal of Pathology*, 1998 153, 271-278.

Liu, YN; Lee, WW; Wang, CY; Chao, TH; Chen, Y; Chen, JH. Regulatory mechanisms controlling human E-cadherin gene expression. *Oncogene*, 2005 24, 8277-8290.

Lo, PK; Mehrotra, J; D'Costa, A; Fackler, MJ; Garrett-Mayer, E; Argani, P; Sukumar, S. Epigenetic suppression of secreted frizzled related protein 1 (SFRP1) expression in human breast cancer. *Cancer Biology and Therapy*, 2006 5, 281-286.

Loeb, DM; Sukumar, S. The role of WT1 in oncogenesis: tumor suppressor or oncogene? *International Journal of Hematology*, 2002 76, 117-126.

Loeb, DM; Evron, E; Patel, CB; Sharma, PM; Niranjan, B; Buluwela, L; Weitzman, SA; Korz, D; Sukumar, S. Wilms' tumor suppressor gene (WT1) is expressed in primary breast tumors despite tumor-specific promoter methylation. *Cancer Research*, 2001 61, 921-925.

Loo, LW; Grove, DI; Williams, EM; Neal, CL; Cousens, LA; Schubert, EL; Holcomb, IN; Massa, HF; Glogovac, J; Li, CI; Malone, KE; Daling, JR; Delrow, JJ; Trask, BJ; Hsu, L; Porter, PL. Array comparative genomic hybridization analysis of genomic alterations in breast cancer subtypes. *Cancer Research*, 2004 64, 8541-8549.

Lucito, R; Healy, J; Alexander, J; Reiner, A; Esposito, D; Chi, M; Rodgers, L; Brady, A; Sebat, J; Troge, J; West, JA; Rostan, S; Nguyen, KC; Powers, S; Ye, KQ; Olshen, A; Venkatraman, E; Norton, L; Wigler, M. Representational oligonucleotide microarray analysis: a high-resolution method to detect genome copy number variation. *Genome Research*, 2003 13, 2291-2305.

Lucke, CD; Philpott, A; Metcalfe, JC; Thompson, AM; Hughes-Davies, L; Kemp, PR; Hesketh, R. Inhibiting mutations in the transforming growth factor beta type 2 receptor in recurrent human breast cancer. *Cancer Research*, 2001 61, 482-485.

Ma, XJ; Salunga, R; Tuggle, JT; Gaudet, J; Enright, E; McQuary, P; Payette, T; Pistone, M; Stecker, K; Zhang, BM; Zhou, YX; Varnholt, H; Smith, B; Gadd, M; Chatfield, E; Kessler, J; Baer, TM; Erlander, MG; Sgroi, DC. Gene expression profiles of human breast cancer progression. *Proceedings of the National Academy of Sciences of the United States of America*, 2003 100, 5974-5979.

Maacke, H; Opitz, S; Jost, K; Hamdorf, W; Henning, W; Kruger, S; Feller, AC; Lopens, A; Diedrich, K; Schwinger, E; Sturzbecher, HW. Over-expression of wild-type Rad51 correlates with histological grading of invasive ductal breast cancer. *International Journal of Cancer*, 2000 88, 907-913.

Maitra, A; Wistuba, II; Washington, C; Virmani, AK; Ashfaq, R; Milchgrub, S; Gazdar, AF; Minna, JD. High-resolution chromosome 3p allelotyping of breast carcinomas and precursor lesions demonstrates frequent loss of heterozygosity and a discontinuous pattern of allele loss. *American Journal of Pathology*, 2001 159, 119-130.

Mao, X; Hamoudi, RA; Zhao, P; Baudis, M. Genetic losses in breast cancer: toward an integrated molecular cytogenetic map. *Cancer Genetics and Cytogenetics*, 2005 160, 141-151.

Martin, ES; Cesari, R; Pentimalli, F; Yoder, K; Fishel, R; Himelstein, AL; Martin, SE; Godwin, AK; Negrini, M; Croce, CM. The BCSC-1 locus at chromosome 11q23-q24 is a candidate tumor suppressor gene. *Proceedings of the National Academy of Sciences of the United States of America*, 2003 100, 11517-11522.

Matsuda, M; Miyagawa, K; Takahashi, M; Fukuda, T; Kataoka, T; Asahara, T; Inui, H; Watatani, M; Yasutomi, M; Kamada, N; Dohi, K; Kamiya, K. Mutations in the RAD54 recombination gene in primary cancers. *Oncogene*, 1999 18, 3427-3430.

Medeiros, AC; Nagai, MA; Neto, MM; Brentani, RR. Loss of heterozygosity affecting the APC and MCC genetic loci in patients with primary breast carcinomas. *Cancer Epidemiology Biomarkers and Prevention,* 1994 3, 331-333.

Meijers-Heijboer, H; van den Ouweland, A; Klijn, J; Wasielewski, M; de Snoo, A; Oldenburg, R; Hollestelle, A; Houben, M; Crepin, E; van Veghel-Plandsoen, M; Elstrodt, F; van Duijn, C; Bartels, C; Meijers, C; Schutte, M; McGuffog, L; Thompson, D; Easton, D; Sodha, N; Seal, S; Barfoot, R; Mangion, J; Chang-Claude, J; Eccles, D; Eeles, R; Evans, DG; Houlston, R; Murday, V; Narod, S; Peretz, T; Peto, J; Phelan, C; Zhang, HX; Szabo, C; Devilee, P; Goldgar, D; Futreal, PA; Nathanson, KL; Weber, B; Rahman, N; Stratton, MR. CHEK2-Breast Cancer Consortium. Low penetrance susceptibility to breast cancer due to CHEK2*1100delC in noncarriers of BRCA1 or BRCA2 mutations. *Nature Genetics* 2002 31, 55–59.

Miller, BJ; Wang, D; Krahe, R; Wright, FA. Pooled analysis of loss of heterozygosity in breast cancer: a genome scan provides comparative evidence for multiple tumor suppressors and identifies novel candidate regions. *American Journal of Human Genetics*, 2003 73, 748-767.

Mironov, N; Jansen, LA; Zhu, WB; Aguelon, AM; Reguer, G; Yamasaki, H. A novel sensitive method to detect frameshift mutations in exonic repeat sequences of cancer-related genes. *Carcinogenesis*, 1999 20, 2189-2192.

Miyoshi, Y; Ando, A; Egawa, C; Taguchi, T; Tamaki, Y; Tamaki, H; Sugiyama, H; Noguchi, S. High expression of Wilms' tumor suppressor gene predicts poor prognosis in breast cancer patients. *Clinical Cancer Research*, 2002 8, 1167-1171.

Mok, SC; Chan, WY; Wong, KK; Cheung, KK; Lau, CC; Ng, SW; Baldini, A; Colitti, CV; Rock, CO; Berkowitz, RS. DOC-2, a candidate tumor suppressor gene in human epithelial ovarian cancer. *Oncogene*, 1998 16, 2381-2387.

Monaco, C; Negrini, M; Sozzi, G; Veronese, ML; Vorechovsky, I; Godwin, AK; Croce, CM. Molecular cloning and characterization of LOH11CR2A, a new gene within a refined minimal region of LOH at 11q23. *Genomics*, 1997 46, 217-222.

Morinaga, N; Shitara, Y; Yanagita, Y; Koida, T; Kimura, M; Asao, T; Kimijima, I; Takenoshita, S; Hirota, T; Saya, H; Kuwano, H. Molecular analysis of the h-warts/LATS1 gene in human breast cancer. *International Journal of Oncology*, 2000 17, 1125-1129.

Mourtada-Maarabouni, M; Keen, J; Clark, J; Cooper, CS; Williams, GT. Candidate tumor suppressor LUCA-15/RBM5/H37 modulates expression of apoptosis and cell cycle genes. *Experimental Cell Research*, 2006 312, 1745-1752.

Munot, K; Bell, SM; Lane, S; Horgan, K; Hanby, AM; Speirs, V. Pattern of expression of genes linked to epigenetic silencing in human breast cancer. *Human Pathology*, 2006 37, 989-999.

Naylor, TL; Greshock, J; Wang, Y; Colligon, T; Yu, QC; Clemmer, V; Zaks, TZ; Weber, BL. High resolution genomic analysis of sporadic breast cancer using array-based comparative genomic hybridization. *Breast Cancer Research*, 2005 7, R1186-R1198.

Nevanlinna, H; Bartek, J. The CHEK2 gene and inherited breast cancer susceptibility. *Oncogene*, 2006 25, 5912-5919.

Nieto, M; Barradas, M; Criado, LM; Flores, JM; Serrano, M; Llano, E. Normal cellular senescence and cancer susceptibility in mice genetically deficient in Ras-induced senescence-1 (Ris1). *Oncogene*, 2006 Sep 11; [Epub ahead of print].

Nobukuni, Y; Kohno, K; Miyagawa, K. Gene trap mutagenesis-based forward genetic approach reveals that the tumor suppressor OVCA1 is a component of the biosynthetic pathway of diphthamide on elongation factor 2. *Journal of Biological Chemistry*, 2005 280, 10572-10577.

Nouet, S; Amzallag, N; Li, JM; Louis, S; Seitz, I; Cui, TX; Alleaume, AM; Di Benedetto, M; Boden, C; Masson, M; Strosberg, AD; Horiuchi, M; Couraud, PO; Nahmias, C. Trans-inactivation of receptor tyrosine kinases by novel angiotensin II AT2 receptor-interacting protein, ATIP. *Journal of Biological Chemistry*, 2004 279, 28989-28997.

Noviello, C; Courjal, F; Theillet, C. Loss of heterozygosity on the long arm of chromosome 6 in breast cancer: possibly four regions of deletion. *Clinical Cancer Research*, 1996 2, 1601-1606.

Nozawa, H; Oda, E; Ueda, S; Tamura, G; Maesawa, C; Muto, T; Taniguchi, T; Tanaka N. Functionally inactivating point mutation in the tumor-suppressor IRF-1 gene identified in human gastric cancer. *International Journal of Cancer*, 1998 77, 522-527.

Oates, AJ; Schumaker, LM; Jenkins, SB; Pearce, AA; DaCosta, SA; Arun, B; Ellis, MJ. The mannose 6-phosphate/insulin-like growth factor 2 receptor (M6P/IGF2R), a putative breast tumor suppressor gene. *Breast Cancer Research and Treatment*, 1998 47, 269-281.

Oh, JJ; West, AR; Fishbein, MC; Slamon, DJ. A candidate tumor suppressor gene, H37, from the human lung cancer tumor suppressor locus 3p21.3. *Cancer Research*, 2002 62, 3207-3213.

Olivier, M; Eeles, R; Hollstein, M; Khan, MA; Harris, CC; Hainaut, P. The IARC TP53 Database: new online mutation analysis and recommendations to users. *Human Mutation*, 2002 19, 607-614.

Osada, H; Tatematsu, Y; Sugito, N; Horio, Y; Takahashi, T. Histone modification in the TGFbetaRII gene promoter and its significance for responsiveness to HDAC inhibitor in lung cancer cell lines. *Molecular Carcinogenesis*, 2005 44, 233-241.

Pal, S; Vishwanath, SN; Erdjument-Bromage, H; Tempst, P; Sif, S. Human SWI/SNF-associated PRMT5 methylates histone H3 arginine 8 and negatively regulates expression of ST7 and NM23 tumor suppressor genes. *Molecular and Cellular Biology*, 2004 24, 9630-9645.

Palamarchuk, A; Efanov, A; Maximov, V; Aqeilan, RI; Croce, CM; Pekarsky Y. Akt phosphorylates and regulates Pdcd4 tumor suppressor protein. *Cancer Research*, 2005 65, 11282-11286.

Panagopoulos, I; Pandis, N; Thelin, S; Petersson, C; Mertens, F; Borg, A; Kristoffersson, U; Mitelman, F; Aman, P. The FHIT and PTPRG genes are deleted in benign proliferative breast disease associated with familial breast cancer and cytogenetic rearrangements of chromosome band 3p14. *Cancer Research*, 1996 56, 4871-4875.

Parrella, P; Scintu, M; Prencipe, M; Poeta, ML; Gallo, AP; Rabitti, C; Rinaldi, M; Tommasi, S; Paradiso, A; Schittulli, F; Valori, VM; Toma, S; Altomare, V; Fazio, VM. HIC1 promoter methylation and 17p13.3 allelic loss in invasive ductal carcinoma of the breast. *Cancer Letters*, 2005 222, 75-81.

Pattingre, S; Levine, B. Bcl-2 inhibition of autophagy: a new route to cancer? *Cancer Research*, 2006 66, 2885-2888.

Peinado, H; Portillo, F; Cano, A. Transcriptional regulation of cadherins during development and carcinogenesis. *International Journal of Developmental Biology*, 2004 48, 365-375.

Peng, H; Xu, F; Pershad, R; Hunt, KK; Frazier, ML; Berchuck, A; Gray, JW; Hogg, D; Bast RC, Jr; Yu Y. ARHI is the center of allelic deletion on chromosome 1p31 in ovarian and breast cancers. *International Journal of Cancer*, 2000 86, 690-694.

Perren, A; Weng, LP; Boag, AH; Ziebold, U; Thakore, K; Dahia, PL; Komminoth, P; Lees, JA; Mulligan, LM; Mutter, GL; Eng, C. Immunohistochemical evidence of loss of PTEN expression in primary ductal adenocarcinomas of the breast. *American Journal of Pathology*, 1999 155, 1253-1260.

Petrocca, F; Iliopoulos, D; Qin, HR; Nicoloso, MS; Yendamuri, S; Wojcik, SE; Shimizu, M; Di Leva, G; Vecchione, A; Trapasso, F; Godwin, AK; Negrini, M; Calin, GA; Croce, CM. Alterations of the Tumor Suppressor Gene ARLTS1 in Ovarian Cancer. *Cancer Research* 2006 66, 10287-10291.

Phelan, CM; Larsson, C; Baird, S; Futreal, PA; Ruttledge, MH; Morgan, K; Tonin, P; Hung, H; Korneluk, RG; Pollak, MN; Narod, SA. The human mammary-derived growth inhibitor (MDGI) gene: genomic structure and mutation analysis in human breast tumors. *Genomics*, 1996 34, 63-68.

Pinte, S; Stankovic-Valentin, N; Deltour, S; Rood, BR; Guerardel, C; Leprince, D. The tumor suppressor gene HIC1 (hypermethylated in cancer 1) is a sequence-specific transcriptional repressor: definition of its consensus binding sequence and analysis of its DNA binding and repressive properties. *Journal of Biological Chemistry*, 2004 279, 38313-38324.

Plaumann, M; Seitz, S; Frege, R; Estevez-Schwarz, L; Scherneck, S. Analysis of DLC-1 expression in human breast cancer. *Journal of Cancer Research and Clinical Oncology*, 2003 129, 349-354.

Pluciennik, E; Kusinska, R; Potemski, P; Kubiak, R; Kordek, R; Bednarek, AK. WWOX--the FRA16D cancer gene: expression correlation with breast cancer progression and prognosis. *European Journal of Surgical Oncology*, 2006 32, 153-157.

Polakis, P. The adenomatous polyposis coli (APC) tumor suppressor. *Biochimica et Biophysica Acta*, 1997 1332, F127-F147.

Powell, JA; Gardner, AE; Bais, AJ; Hinze, SJ; Baker, E; Whitmore, S; Crawford, J; Kochetkova, M; Spendlove, HE; Doggett, NA; Sutherland, GR; Callen, DF; Kremmidiotis, G. Sequencing, transcript identification, and quantitative gene expression profiling in the breast cancer loss of heterozygosity region 16q24.3 reveal three potential tumor-suppressor genes. *Genomics*, 2002 80, 303-310.

Powell, SN; Kachnic, LA. Roles of BRCA1 and BRCA2 in homologous recombination, DNA replication fidelity and the cellular response to ionizing radiation. *Oncogene*, 2003 22, 5784-5791.

Qu, X; Yu, J; Bhagat, G; Furuya, N; Hibshoosh, H; Troxel, A; Rosen, J; Eskelinen, EL; Mizushima, N; Ohsumi, Y; Cattoretti, G; Levine B. Promotion of tumorigenesis by heterozygous disruption of the beclin 1 autophagy gene. *Clinical Investigations*, 2003 112, 1809-1820.

Raderschall, E; Stout, K; Freier, S; Suckow, V; Schweiger, S; Haaf, T. Elevated levels of Rad51 recombination protein in tumor cells. *Cancer Research*, 2002 62, 219-225.

Rai, R; Dai, H; Multani, AS; Li, K; Chin, K; Gray, J; Lahad, JP; Liang, J; Mills, GB; Meric-Bernstam, F; Lin, SY. BRIT1 regulates early DNA damage response, chromosomal integrity, and cancer. *Cancer Cell*, 2006 10, 145-57.

Rakha, EA; Putti, TC; Abd El-Rehim, DM; Paish, C; Green, AR; Powe, DG; Lee, AH; Robertson, JF; Ellis, IO. Morphological and immunophenotypic analysis of breast carcinomas with basal and myoepithelial differentiation. *Journal of Pathology*, 2006 208, 495-506.

Rasio, D; Murakumo, Y; Robbins, D; Roth, T; Silver, A; Negrini, M; Schmidt, C; Burczak, J; Fishel, R; Croce, CM. Characterization of the human homologue of RAD54: a gene located on chromosome 1p32 at a region of high loss of heterozygosity in breast tumors. *Cancer Research*, 1997 57, 2378-2383.

Renwick, A; Thompson, D; Seal, S; Kelly, P; Chagtai, T; Ahmed, M; North, B; Jayatilake, H; Barfoot, R; Spanova, K; McGuffog, L; Evans, DG; Eccles, D; Breast Cancer Susceptibility Collaboration; Easton, DF; Stratton, MR; Rahman N. ATM mutations that cause ataxia-telangiectasia are breast cancer susceptibility alleles. *Nature Genetics*, 2006 38, 873-875.

Rintala-Maki, ND; Abrasonis, V; Burd, M; Sutherland, LC. Genetic instability of RBM5/LUCA-15/H37 in MCF-7 breast carcinoma sublines may affect susceptibility to apoptosis. *Cell Biochemistry and Function*, 2004 22, 307-313.

Ristimaki, A; Sivula, A; Lundin, J; Lundin, M; Salminen, T; Haglund, C; Joensuu, H; Isola, J. Prognostic significance of elevated cyclooxygenase-2 expression in breast cancer. *Cancer Research*, 2002 62, 632-635.

Rivenbark, AG; Jones, WD; Coleman WB. DNA methylation-dependent silencing of CST6 in human breast cancer cell lines. *Laboratory Investigations*, 2006 Oct 16; [Epub ahead of print].

Roberts, CW; Leroux, MM; Fleming, MD; Orkin, SH. Highly penetrant, rapid tumorigenesis through conditional inversion of the tumor suppressor gene Snf5. *Cancer Cell*, 2002 2, 415-425.

Rosen, EM; Fan, S; Pestell, RG; Goldberg, ID. BRCA1 gene in breast cancer. *Journal of Cell Physiology*, 2003 196, 19-41.

Rosner, M; Freilinger, A; Hengstschlager, M. The tuberous sclerosis genes and regulation of the cyclin-dependent kinase inhibitor p27. *Mutation Research*, 2006 613, 10-16.

Rowan, A; Churchman, M; Jefferey, R; Hanby, A; Poulsom, R; Tomlinson, I. In situ analysis of LKB1/STK11 mRNA expression in human normal tissues and tumours. *Journal of Pathology*, 2000 192, 203-206.

Sansal, I; Sellers, WR. The biology and clinical relevance of the PTEN tumor suppressor pathway. *Journal of Clinical Oncology*, 2004 22, 2954-2963.

Sarrio, D; Moreno-Bueno, G; Hardisson, D; Sanchez-Estevez, C; Guo, M; Herman, JG; Gamallo, C; Esteller, M; Palacios, J. Epigenetic and genetic alterations of APC and CDH1 genes in lobular breast cancer: relationships with abnormal E-cadherin and catenin expression and microsatellite instability. *International Journal of Cancer*, 2003 106, 208-215.

Savino, M; d'Apolito, M; Centra, M; van Beerendonk, HM; Cleton-Jansen, AM; Whitmore, SA; Crawford, J; Callen, DF; Zelante, L; Savoia A. Characterization of copine VII, a new member of the copine family, and its exclusion as a candidate in sporadic breast cancers with loss of heterozygosity at 16q24.3. *Genomics*, 1999 61, 219-226.

Schenk, M; Leib-Mosch, C; Schenck, IU; Jaenicke, M; Indraccolo, S; Saeger, HD; Dallenbach-Hellweg, G; Hehlmann R. Lower frequency of allele loss on chromosome 18q in human breast cancer than in colorectal tumors. *Journal of Molecular Medicine*, 1996 74, 155-159.

Schmutte, C; Tombline, G; Rhiem, K; Sadoff, MM; Schmutzler, R; von Deimling, A; Fishel, R. Characterization of the human Rad51 genomic locus and examination of tumors with 15q14-15 loss of heterozygosity (LOH). *Cancer Research* 1999 59, 4564-4569.

Schultz, DC; Vanderveer, L; Berman, DB; Hamilton, TC; Wong, AJ; Godwin, AK. Identification of two candidate tumor suppressor genes on chromosome 17p13.3. *Cancer Research*, 1996 56, 1997-2002.

Schutte, M; Hruban, RH; Hedrick, L; Cho, KR; Nadasdy, GM; Weinstein, CL; Bova, GS; Isaacs, WB; Cairns, P; Nawroz, H; Sidransky, D; Casero, RA Jr; Meltzer, PS; Hahn, SA; Kern SE. DPC4 gene in various tumor types. *Cancer Research*, 1996 56, 2527-2530.

Schutte, M; Seal, S; Barfoot, R; Meijers-Heijboer, H; Wasielewski, M; Evans, DG; Eccles, D; Meijers, C; Lohman, F; Klijn, J; van den Ouweland, A; Futreal, PA; Nathanson, KL; Weber, BL; Easton, DF; Stratton, MR; Rahman, N; Breast Cancer Linkage Consortium. Variants in CHEK2 other than 1100delC do not make a major contribution to breast cancer susceptibility. *American Journal of Human Genetics*, 2003 72, 1023-1028.

Seitz, S; Poppe, K; Fischer, J; Nothnagel, A; Estevez-Schwarz, L; Haensch, W; Schlag, PM; Scherneck, S. Detailed deletion mapping in sporadic breast cancer at chromosomal region 17p13 distal to the TP53 gene: association with clinicopathological parameters. *Journal of Pathology*, 2001 194, 318-326.

Sekine, I; Sato, M; Sunaga, N; Toyooka, S; Peyton, M; Parsons, R; Wang, W; Gazdar, AF; Minna, JD. The 3p21 candidate tumor suppressor gene BAF180 is normally expressed in human lung cancer. *Oncogene*, 2005 24, 2735-2738.

Senchenko, V; Liu, J; Braga, E; Mazurenko, N; Loginov, W; Seryogin, Y; Bazov, I; Protopopov, A; Kisseljov, FL; Kashuba, V; Lerman, MI; Klein, G; Zabarovsky, ER. Deletion mapping using quantitative real-time PCR identifies two distinct 3p21.3 regions affected in most cervical carcinomas. *Oncogene*, 2003 22 2984-2992.

Senchenko, VN; Liu, J; Loginov, W; Bazov, I; Angeloni, D; Seryogin, Y; Ermilova, V; Kazubskaya, T; Garkavtseva, R; Zabarovska, VI; Kashuba, VI; Kisselev, LL; Minna, JD; Lerman, MI; Klein, G; Braga, EA; Zabarovsky, ER. Discovery of frequent homozygous deletions in chromosome 3p21.3 LUCA and AP20 regions in renal, lung and breast carcinomas. *Oncogene* 2004 23, 5719-5728.

Sevignani, C; Calin, GA; Cesari, R; Sarti, M; Ishii, H; Yendamuri, S; Vecchione, A; Trapasso, F; Croce, CM. Restoration of fragile histidine triad (FHIT) expression induces apoptosis and suppresses tumorigenicity in breast cancer cell lines. *Cancer Research*, 2003 63 1183-1187.

Sharpless, NE; DePinho, RA. The INK4A/ARF locus and its two gene products. *Current Opinion in Genetics and Development*, 1999 9, 22-30.

Sharpless, NE. INK4a/ARF: a multifunctional tumor suppressor locus. *Mutation Research*, 2005 576, 22-38.

Shen, Z; Wen, XF; Lan, F; Shen, ZZ; Shao, ZM. The tumor suppressor gene LKB1 is associated with prognosis in human breast carcinoma. *Clinical Cancer Research*, 2002 8, 2085-2090.

Sherr, CJ; Weber, JD. The ARF/p53 pathway. *Current Opinion in Genetics and Development*, 2000 10, 94-99.

Shinozaki, M; Hoon, DS; Giuliano, AE; Hansen, NM; Wang, HJ; Turner, R; Taback, B. Distinct hypermethylation profile of primary breast cancer is associated with sentinel lymph node metastasis. *Clinical Cancer Research*, 2005 11, 2156-2162.

Shivapurkar, N; Sood, S; Wistuba, II; Virmani, AK; Maitra, A; Milchgrub, S; Minna, JD; Gazdar, AF. Multiple regions of chromosome 4 demonstrating allelic losses in breast carcinomas. *Cancer Research*, 1999 59, 3576-3580.

Silva, J; Silva, JM; Dominguez, G; Garcia, JM; Cantos, B; Rodriguez, R; Larrondo, FJ; Provencio, M; Espana, P; Bonilla, F. Concomitant expression of p16INK4a and p14ARF in primary breast cancer and analysis of inactivation mechanisms. *Journal of Pathology*, 2003 199, 289-297.

Silva, J; Silva, JM; Barradas, M; Garcia, JM; Dominguez, G; Garcia, V; Pena, C; Gallego, I; Espinosa, R; Serrano, M; Bonilla, F. Analysis of the candidate tumor suppressor Ris-1 in primary human breast carcinomas. *Mutation Research*, 2006 594, 78-85.

Simpson, PT ; Gale, T ; Reis-Filho, JS; Jones, C; Parry, S; Steele, D; Cossu, A; Budroni, M; Palmieri, G; Lakhani, SR. Distribution and significance of 14–3-3sigma, a novel myoepithelial marker, in normal, benign, and malignant breast tissue. *Journal of Pathology*, 2004 202, 274–285.

Sirchia, SM; Ferguson, AT; Sironi, E; Subramanyan, S; Orlandi, R; Sukumar, S; Sacchi, N. Evidence of epigenetic changes affecting the chromatin state of the retinoic acid receptor beta2 promoter in breast cancer cells. *Oncogene,* 2000 19, 1556-1563.

Siripurapu, V; Meth, J; Kobayashi, N; Hamaguchi, M. DBC2 significantly influences cell-cycle, apoptosis, cytoskeleton and membrane-trafficking pathways. *Journal of Molecular Biology*, 2005 346, 83-89.

Sodha, N; Bullock, S; Taylor, R; Mitchell, G; Guertl-Lackner, B; Williams, RD; Bevan, S; Bishop, K; McGuire, S; Houlston, RS; Eeles, RA. CHEK2 variants in susceptibility to breast cancer and evidence of retention of the wild type allele in tumours. *British Journal of Cancer*, 2002 87, 1445-1448.

Song, J; Jie, C; Polk, P; Shridhar, R; Clair, T; Zhang, J; Yin, L; Keppler, D. The candidate tumor suppressor CST6 alters the gene expression profile of human breast carcinoma cells: down-regulation of the potent mitogenic, motogenic, and angiogenic factor autotaxin. *Biochemical and Biophysical Research Communications*, 2006 340, 175-182.

Sourvinos, G; Miyakis, S; Liloglou, TL; Field, JK; Spandidos, DA. Von Hippel-Lindau tumour suppressor gene is not involved in sporadic human breast cancer. *Tumour Biology*, 2001 22, 131-6.

Staalesen, V; Falck, J; Geisler, S; Bartkova, J; Borresen-Dale, AL; Lukas, J; Lillehaug, JR; Bartek, J; Lonning, PE. Alternative splicing and mutation status of CHEK2 in stage III breast cancer. *Oncogene*, 2004 23, 8535-8544.

Starita, LM; Parvin, JD. The multiple nuclear functions of BRCA1: transcription, ubiquitination and DNA repair. *Current Opinion in Cell Biology*, 2003 15, 345-350.

Stemmer-Rachamimov, AO; Wiederhold, T; Nielsen, GP; James, M; Pinney-Michalowski, D; Roy, JE; Cohen, WA; Ramesh, V; Louis, DN. NHE-RF, a merlin-interacting protein, is primarily expressed in luminal epithelia, proliferative endometrium, and estrogen receptor-positive breast carcinomas. *American Journal of Pathology*, 2001 158, 57-62.

Sterling, JA; Wu, L; Banerji, SS. PARP regulates TGF-beta receptor type II expression in estrogen receptor-positive breast cancer cell lines. *Anticancer Research*, 2006 26 1893-1901.

Stuelten, CH; Buck, MB; Dippon, J; Roberts, AB; Fritz, P; Knabbe, C. Smad4-expression is decreased in breast cancer tissues: a retrospective study. *BMC Cancer*, 2006 6, 25.

Su, GH; Hilgers, W; Shekher, MC; Tang, DJ; Yeo, CJ; Hruban, RH; Kern, SE. Alterations in pancreatic, biliary, and breast carcinomas support MKK4 as a genetically targeted tumor suppressor gene. *Cancer Research*, 1998 58, 2339-2342.

Su, G ; Roberts, T ; Cowell, JK. TTC4, a novel human gene containing the tetratricopeptide repeat and mapping to the region of chromosome 1p31 that is frequently deleted in sporadic breast cancer. *Genomics*, 1999 55, 157-163.

Su, G; Casey, G; Cowell, JK. Genomic structure of the human tetratricopeptide repeat-containing gene, TTC4, from chromosome region 1p31 and mutation analysis in breast cancers. *International Journal of Molecular Medicine*, 2000 5, 197-200.

Su, GH; Song, JJ; Repasky, EA; Schutte, M; Kern, SE. Mutation rate of MAP2K4/MKK4 in breast carcinoma. *Human Mutation*, 2002 19, 81.

Sugimura, J; Tamura, G; Suzuki, Y; Fujioka, T. Allelic loss on chromosomes 3p, 5q and 17p in renal cell carcinomas. *Pathology International*, 1997 47, 79-83.

Sullivan, A; Yuille, M; Repellin, C; Reddy, A; Reelfs, O; Bell, A; Dunne, B; Gusterson, BA; Osin, P; Farrell, PJ; Yulug, I; Evans, A; Ozcelik, T; Gasco, M; Crook, T. Concomitant inactivation of p53 and Chk2 in breast cancer. *Oncogene*, 2002 21, 1316-1324.

Sun, X; Zhou, Y; Otto, KB; Wang, M; Chen, C; Zhou, W; Subramanian, K; Vertino, PM; Dong, JT. Infrequent mutation of ATBF1 in human breast cancer. *Journal of Cancer Research and Clinical Oncology*, 2006 Aug 24; [Epub ahead of print].

Sundaresan, V; Chung, G; Heppell-Parton, A; Xiong, J; Grundy, C; Roberts, I; James, L; Cahn, A; Bench, A; Douglas, J; Minna, J; Sekido, Y; Lerman, M; Latif, F; Bergh, J; Li, H; Lowe, N; Ogilvie, D; Rabbitts, P. Homozygous deletions at 3p12 in breast and lung cancer. *Oncogene*, 1998 17, 1723-1729.

Takahashi, Y; Miyoshi, Y; Takahata, C; Irahara, N; Taguchi, T; Tamaki, Y; Noguchi, S. Down-regulation of LATS1 and LATS2 mRNA expression by promoter hypermethylation and its association with biologically aggressive phenotype in human breast cancers. *Clinical Cancer Research*, 2005 11, 1380-1385.

Takenoshita, S; Mogi, A; Tani, M; Osawa, H; Sunaga, H; Kakegawa, H; Yanagita, Y; Koida, T; Kimura, M; Fujita, KI; Kato, H; Kato, R; Nagamachi, Y. Absence of mutations in the analysis of coding sequences of the entire transforming growth factor-beta type II receptor gene in sporadic human breast cancers. *Oncology Reports*, 1998 5, 367-371.

Tang, K; Oeth, P; Kammerer, S; Denissenko, MF; Ekblom, J; Jurinke, C; van den Boom, D; Braun, A; Cantor CR. Mining disease susceptibility genes through SNP analyses and expression profiling using MALDI-TOF mass spectrometry. *Journal of Proteome Research*, 2004 3, 218-227.

Teng, DH; Perry, WL 3rd; Hogan, JK; Baumgard, M; Bell, R; Berry, S; Davis, T; Frank, D; Frye, C; Hattier, T; Hu, R; Jammulapati, S; Janecki, T; Leavitt, A; Mitchell, JT; Pero, R; Sexton, D; Schroeder, M; Su, PH; Swedlund, B; Kyriakis, JM; Avruch, J; Bartel, P; Wong, AK; Tavtigian, SV, et al. Human mitogen-activated protein kinase kinase 4 as a candidate tumor suppressor. *Cancer Research*, 1997 57, 4177-4182.

Theile, M; Seitz, S; Arnold, W; Jandrig, B; Frege, R; Schlag, PM; Haensch, W; Guski, H; Winzer, KJ; Barrett, JC; Scherneck S. A defined chromosome 6q fragment (at D6S310) harbors a putative tumor suppressor gene for breast cancer. *Oncogene*, 1996 13, 677-685.

Thomas, NA; Choong, DY; Jokubaitis, VJ; Neville, PJ; Campbell, IG. Mutation of the ST7 tumor suppressor gene on 7q31.1 is rare in breast, ovarian and colorectal cancers. *Nature Genetics*, 2001 29, 379-380.

Tirkkonen, M; Tanner, M; Karhu, R; Kallioniemi, A; Isola, J; Kallioniemi, OP. Molecular cytogenetics of primary breast cancer by CGH. *Genes Chromosomes and Cancer*, 1998 21, 177-184.

Tomizawa, Y; Sekido, Y; Kondo, M; Gao, B; Yokota, J; Roche, J; Drabkin, H; Lerman, MI; Gazdar, AF; Minna, JD. Inhibition of lung cancer cell growth and induction of apoptosis after reexpression of 3p21.3 candidate tumor suppressor gene SEMA3B. *Proceedings of the National Academy of Sciences of the United States of America*, 2001 98, 13954-13959.

van Wezel, T; Lombaerts, M; van Roon, EH; Philippo, K; Baelde, HJ; Szuhai, K; Cornelisse, CJ; Cleton-Jansen, AM. Expression analysis of candidate breast tumour suppressor genes on chromosome 16q. *Breast Cancer Research*, 2005 7, R998-R1004.

van 't Veer, LJ; Dai, H; van de Vijver, MJ; He, YD; Hart, AA; Mao, M; Peterse, HL; van der Kooy, K; Marton, MJ; Witteveen, AT; Schreiber, GJ; Kerkhoven, RM; Roberts, C; Linsley, PS; Bernards, R; Friend, SH. Gene expression profiling predicts clinical outcome of breast cancer. *Nature*, 2002 415, 530-536.

Vecchione, A; Ishii, H; Shiao, YH; Trapasso, F; Rugge, M; Tamburrino, JF; Murakumo, Y; Alder, H; Croce, CM; Baffa R. Fez1/lzts1 alterations in gastric carcinoma. *Clinical Cancer Research*, 2001 7, 1546-1552.

Veeck, J; Niederacher, D; An, H; Klopocki, E; Wiesmann, F; Betz, B; Galm, O; Camara, O; Durst, M; Kristiansen, G; Huszka, C; Knuchel, R; Dahl, E. Aberrant methylation of the Wnt antagonist SFRP1 in breast cancer is associated with unfavourable prognosis. *Oncogene*, 2006 25, 3479-3488.

Venter, DJ; Ramus, SJ; Hammet, FM; de Silva, M; Hutchins, AM; Petrovic, V; Price, G; Armes, JE. Complex CGH alterations on chromosome arm 8p at candidate tumor suppressor gene loci in breast cancer cell lines. *Cancer Genetics and Cytogenetics,* 2005 160, 134-140.

Vestey SB, Sen C, Calder CJ, Perks CM, Pignatelli M, Winters ZE. p14ARF expression in invasive breast cancers and ductal carcinoma in situ--relationships to p53 and Hdm2. *Breast Cancer Research*, 2004 6, R571-R585.

Virmani, AK; Rathi, A; Sathyanarayana, UG; Padar, A; Huang, CX; Cunnigham, HT; Farinas, AJ; Milchgrub; Euhus, DM; Gilcrease, M; Herman, J; Minna, JD; Gazdar, AF. Aberrant methylation of the adenomatous polyposis coli (APC) gene promoter 1A in breast and lung carcinomas. *Clinical Cancer Research*, 2001 7, 1998-2004.

Wagner, KU; Krempler, A; Qi, Y; Park, K; Henry, MD; Triplett, AA; Riedlinger, G; Rucker, III EB; Hennighausen, L. Tsg101 is essential for cell growth, proliferation, and cell survival of embryonic and adult tissues. *Molecular and Cellular Biology*, 2003 23, 150-162.

Wales, MM; Biel, MA; el Deiry, W; Nelkin, BD; Issa, JP; Cavenee, WK; Kuerbitz, SJ; Baylin, SB. p53 activates expression of HIC-1, a new candidate tumour suppressor gene on 17p13.3. *Nature Medicine*, 1995 1, 570-577.

Wang, H; Bedford, FK; Brandon, NJ; Moss, SJ; Olsen, RW. GABA(A)-receptor-associated protein links GABA(A) receptors and the cytoskeleton. *Nature*, 1999 397, 69-72.

Wang, Z; Tseng, CP; Pong, RC; Chen, H; McConnell, JD; Navone, N; Hsieh, JT. The mechanism of growth-inhibitory effect of DOC-2/DAB2 in prostate cancer. *Journal of Biological Chemistry*, 2002 277, 12622-12631.

Wang, N; Leeming, R; Abdul-Karim, FW. Fine needle aspiration cytology of breast cylindroma in a woman with familial cylindromatosis: a case report. *Acta Cytologica*, 2004a 48, 853-858.

Wang, L; Pan, Y; Dai, JL. Evidence of MKK4 pro-oncogenic activity in breast and pancreatic tumors. *Oncogene* 2004b 23, 5978-5985.

Wang, Y; Klijn, JG; Zhang, Y; Sieuwerts, AM; Look, MP; Yang, F; Talantov, D; Timmermans, M; Meijer-van Gelder, ME; Yu, J; Jatkoe, T; Berns, EM; Atkins, D; Foekens, JA. Gene-expression profiles to predict distant metastasis of lymph-node-negative primary breast cancer. *Lancet*, 2005a 365, 671-679.

Wang, L; Devarajan, E; He, J; Reddy, SP; Dai, JL. Transcription repressor activity of spleen tyrosine kinase mediates breast tumor suppression. *Cancer Research*, 2005b 65, 10289-10297.

Wang, LS; Huang, YW; Sugimoto, Y; Liu, S; Chang, HL; Ye, W; Shu, S; Lin, YC. Conjugated linoleic acid (CLA) up-regulates the estrogen-regulated cancer suppressor gene, protein tyrosine phosphatase gamma (PTPgamma), in human breast cells. *Anticancer Research*, 2006a 26, 27-34.

Wang, HC; Chou, WC; Shieh, SY; Shen CY. Ataxia telangiectasia mutated and checkpoint kinase 2 regulate BRCA1 to promote the fidelity of DNA end-joining. *Cancer Research*, 2006 66, 1391-1400.

Watanabe, A; Hippo, Y; Taniguchi, H; Iwanari, H; Yashiro, M; Hirakawa, K; Kodama, T; Aburatani, H. An opposing view on WWOX protein function as a tumor suppressor. *Cancer Research*, 2003 63, 8629-8633.

Wei, C; Amos, CI; Stephens, LC; Campos, I; Deng, JM; Behringer, RR; Rashid, A; Frazier, ML. Mutation of Lkb1 and p53 genes exert a cooperative effect on tumorigenesis. *Cancer Research*, 2005 65, 11297-11303.

Weischer, M; Bojesen, SE; Tybjaerg-Hansen, A; Axelsson, CK; Nordestgaard, BG. Increased Risk of Breast Cancer Associated With CHEK2*1100delC. *Journal of Clinical Oncology*, 2006 Jul 31; [Epub ahead of print].

Weith, A; Brodeur, GM; Bruns, GA; Matise, TC; Mischke, D; Nizetic, D; Seldin, MF; van Roy, N; Vance, J. Report of the second international workshop on human chromosome 1 mapping 1995. *Cytogenetics and Cell Genetics*, 1996 72, 114-144.

Welcsh, PL; King, MC. BRCA1 and BRCA2 and the genetics of breast and ovarian cancer. *Human Molecular Genetics*, 2001 10, 705-713.

White, GR; Varley, JM; Heighway, J. Genomic structure and expression profile of LPHH1, a 7TM gene variably expressed in breast cancer cell lines. *Biochimica et Biophysica Acta*, 2000 1491, 85-92.

Whitmore, SA; Settasatian, C; Crawford, J; Lower, KM; McCallum, B; Seshadri, R; Cornelisse, CJ; Moerland, EW; Cleton-Jansen, AM; Tipping, AJ; Mathew, CG; Savnio, M; Savoia, A; Verlander, P; Auerbach, AD; Van Berkel, C; Pronk, JC; Doggett, NA; Callen, DF. Characterization and screening for mutations of the growth arrest-specific 11 (GAS11) and C16orf3 genes at 16q24.3 in breast cancer. *Genomics*, 1998 52, 325-331.

Wick, W; Petersen, I; Schmutzler, RK; Wolfarth, B; Lenartz, D; Bierhoff, E; Hummerich, J; Muller, DJ; Stangl, AP; Schramm, J; Wiestler, OD; von Deimling, A. Evidence for a novel tumor suppressor gene on chromosome 15 associated with progression to a metastatic stage in breast cancer. *Oncogene*, 1996 12, 973-978.

Wilentz, RE; Argani, P; Hruban, RH. Loss of heterozygosity or intragenic mutation, which comes first? *American Journal of Pathology*, 2001 158, 1561–1563.

Wolf, I; O'Kelly, J; Rubinek, T; Tong, M; Nguyen, A; Lin, BT; Tai, HH; Karlan, BY; Koeffler, HP. 15-hydroxyprostaglandin dehydrogenase is a tumor suppressor of human breast cancer. *Cancer Research*, 2006 66, 7818-7823.

Wu, X; Webster, SR; Chen, J. Characterization of tumor-associated Chk2 mutations. *Journal of Biological Chemistry*, 2001 276, 2971–2974.

Xie, D; Jauch, A; Miller, CW; Bartram, CR; Koeffler, HP. Discovery of over-expressed genes and genetic alterations in breast cancer cells using a combination of suppression subtractive hybridization, multiplex FISH and comparative genomic hybridization. *International Journal of Oncology*, 2002 21, 499-507.

Yaegashi, S; Sachse, R; Ohuchi, N; Mori, S; Sekiya, T. Low incidence of a nucleotide sequence alteration of the neurofibromatosis 2 gene in human breast cancers. *Japanese Journal of Cancer Research*, 1995 86, 929-933.

Yang, Q; Nakamura, M; Nakamura, Y; Yoshimura, G; Suzuma, T; Umemura, T; Shimizu, Y; Mori, I; Sakurai, T; Kakudo, K. Two-hit inactivation of FHIT by loss of heterozygosity and hypermethylation in breast cancer. *Clinical Cancer Research*, 2002a 8, 2890-2893.

Yang, Q; Yoshimura, G; Mori, I; Sakurai, T; Kakudo, K. Chromosome 3p and breast cancer. *Journal of Human Genetics* 2002b 47, 453-459.

Yang, TL; Su, YR; Huang, CS; Yu, JC; Lo, YL; Wu, PE; Shen, CY. High-resolution 19p13.2-13.3 allelotyping of breast carcinomas demonstrates frequent loss of heterozygosity. Genes Chromosomes and Cancer, 2004 41, 250-256.

Ylikorkala, A; Avizienyte, E; Tomlinson, IP; Tiainen, M; Roth, S; Loukola, A; Hemminki, A; Johansson, M; Sistonen, P; Markie, D; Neale, K; Phillips, R; Zauber, P; Twama, T; Sampson, J; Jarvinen, H; Makela, TP; Aaltonen, LA. Mutations and impaired function of LKB1 in familial and non-familial Peutz-Jeghers syndrome and a sporadic testicular cancer. *Human Molecular Genetics*, 1999 8, 45-51.

Yokota, T; Matsumoto, S; Yoshimoto, M; Kasumi, F; Akiyama, F; Sakamoto, G; Nakamura, Y; Emi, M. Mapping of a breast cancer tumor suppressor gene locus to a 4-cM interval on chromosome 18q21. *Japan Journal of Cancer Research*, 1997 88, 959-964.

Yoshikawa, K; Ogawa, T; Baer, R; Hemmi, H; Honda, K; Yamauchi, A; Inamoto, T; Ko, K; Yazumi, S; Motoda, H; Kodama, H; Noguchi, S; Gazdar, AF; Yamaoka, Y; Takahashi, R. Abnormal expression of BRCA1 and BRCA1-interactive DNA-repair proteins in breast carcinomas. *International Journal of Cancer*, 2000 88, 28-36.

Yu, Y; Xu, F; Peng, H; Fang, X; Zhao, S; Li, Y; Cuevas, B; Kuo, WL; Gray, JW; Siciliano, M; Mills, GB; Bast, RC Jr. NOEY2 (ARHI), an imprinted putative tumor suppressor gene in ovarian and breast carcinomas. *Proceedings of the National Academy of Sciences of the United States of America,* 1999 96, 214-219.

Yu, TW; Bargmann, CI. Dynamic regulation of axon guidance. *Nature Neurosciences*, 2001 4 Suppl, 1169-1176.

Yu, Y; Fujii, S; Yuan, J; Luo, RZ; Wang, L; Bao, J; Kadota, M; Oshimura, M; Dent, SR; Issa, JP; Bast RC Jr. Epigenetic regulation of ARHI in breast and ovarian cancer cells. *Annals of the New York Academy of Sciences,* 2003 983, 268-277.

Yu, Y; Luo, R; Lu, Z; Wei Feng, W; Badgwell, D; Issa, JP; Rosen, DG; Liu, J; Bast RC Jr. Biochemistry and Biology of ARHI (DIRAS3), an Imprinted Tumor Suppressor Gene Whose Expression Is Lost in Ovarian and Breast Cancers. *Methods in Enzymology,* 2005 407, 455-468.

Yuan, Y; Mendez, R; Sahin, A; Dai, JL. Hypermethylation leads to silencing of the SYK gene in human breast cancer. *Cancer Research*, 2001 61, 5558-5561.

Yuan, BZ; Zhou, X; Durkin, ME; Zimonjic, DB; Gumundsdottir, K; Eyfjord, JE; Thorgeirsson, SS; Popescu NC. DLC-1 gene inhibits human breast cancer cell growth and in vivo tumorigenicity. *Oncogene* 2003 22, 445–450.

Yue, Z; Jin, S; Yang, C; Levine, AJ; Heintz, N. Beclin 1, an autophagy gene essential for early embryonic development, is a haploinsufficient tumor suppressor. *Proceedings of the National Academy of Sciences of the United States of America*, 2003 100, 15077-15082.

Zapata-Benavides, P; Tuna, M; Lopez-Berestein, G; Tari, AM. Downregulation of Wilms' tumor 1 protein inhibits breast cancer proliferation. *Biochemical and Biophysical Research Communications*, 2002 295, 784-790.

Zenklusen, JC; Bieche, I; Lidereau, R; Conti, CJ. (C-A)n microsatellite repeat D7S522 is the most commonly deleted region in human primary breast cancer. *Proceedings of the National Academy of Sciences of the United States of America*, 1994 91, 12155-12158.

Zenklusen, JC; Conti, CJ; Green, ED. Mutational and functional analyses reveal that ST7 is a highly conserved tumor-suppressor gene on human chromosome 7q31. *Nature Genetics*, 2001 27 392-398.

Zhang, TF; Yu, SQ; Guan, LS; Wang, ZY. 2003 Inhibition of breast cancer cell growth by the Wilms' tumor suppressor WT1 is associated with a destabilization of ß-catenin. *Anticancer Research*, 2003 23, 3575–3584.

Zhang, H; Ozaki, I; Mizuta, T; Hamajima, H; Yasutake, T; Eguchi, Y; Ideguchi, H; Yamamoto, K; Matsuhashi S. Involvement of programmed cell death 4 in transforming growth factor-beta1-induced apoptosis in human hepatocellular carcinoma. *Oncogene*, 2006 25, 6101-6112.

Zhong, D; Morikawa, A; Guo, L; Colpaert, C; Xiong, L; Nassar, A; Chen, C; Lamb, N; Dong, JT; Zhou W. Homozygous Deletion of SMAD4 in Breast Cancer Cell Lines and Invasive Ductal Carcinomas. *Cancer Biology and Therapy*, 2006 5, 601-607.

Zhu, G; Gilchrist, R; Borley, N; Chng, HW; Morgan, M; Marshall, JF; Camplejohn, RS; Muir, GH; Hart, IR. Reduction of TSG101 protein has a negative impact on tumor cell growth. *International Journal of Cancer*, 2004 109, 541-547.

INDEX

A

aberrant, 17, 28, 30, 34, 39, 42, 43, 54
aberrant methylation, 30, 42, 43
abnormalities, 24, 53, 59
absorption, 60
access, 62
acetylation, 5, 16
acid, 7, 11, 12, 17, 21, 26, 36, 56, 65, 84, 95, 99
actin, 15, 34, 59, 60
activation, 5, 6, 31, 32, 44, 50, 73, 80
adducts, 41
adenocarcinoma (s), 59, 79, 90
adenoma, 12
Adenomatosis polyposis coli (APC), 12, 30, 87, 91, 93, 98
adenovirus, 13
adhesion, 19, 43, 50
ADP, 14, 47, 58
adult, 26, 60, 98
agar, 17, 35, 37, 42, 56, 59, 63
age, 5, 48
agent (s), 28, 34, 41
aggregation, 27
aggressiveness, 42, 60
alkylation, 41
allele (s), 3, 16, 21, 26, 32, 40, 44, 45, 46, 51, 52, 57, 59, 61, 62, 64, 87, 92, 93, 95

alpha, 11, 14, 16, 22, 61, 73, 86
alternative, 26, 38, 80
alters, 95
Alzheimer's disease, 49
amino, 7, 21, 36, 50, 65
amino acid (s), 7, 50, 65
anaemia, 74
anemia, 13, 14
angiogenesis, 5, 28
angiogenic, 74, 95
angiotensin II, 13, 36, 76, 89
annealing, ix, 10
antagonist, 33, 98
anti-proliferative, 5
anti-tumor, 7, 23
apoptosis, vii, 5, 7, 10, 15, 18, 19, 20, 22, 24, 28, 31, 32, 35, 40, 47, 52, 55, 56, 57, 59, 61, 64, 67, 73, 74, 80, 83, 86, 88, 92, 94, 95, 97, 102
apoptotic, 22, 23, 35, 47, 53
apoptotic pathway, 23
arginine, 33, 90
arrest, 5, 14, 19, 28, 32, 45, 55, 62, 64, 80, 99
aspiration, 98
associations, 53
ataxia, 43, 44, 92
Ataxia telangiectasia mutated (ATM), 1, 6, 9, 13, 27, 43, 44, 47, 64, 71, 72, 85, 92
autism, 48
autophagic cell death, 59
autophagy, 16, 58, 86, 90, 91, 101

autosomal dominant, 9, 30, 48
autosomal recessive, 43
availability, 22
axon, 11, 101
axonal, 24, 27, 61

B

B cell lymphoma, 59
bacterial, 58
base pair, 10, 37, 53
Bcl-2, 53, 59, 90
behavior, 18, 67
benign, 20, 38, 90, 95
beta, 12, 17, 60, 76, 79, 87
bilateral, 47
binding, 7, 11, 12, 14, 15, 17, 22, 37, 50, 64,
    78, 91
biochemical, 39, 56
bioinformatics, 63
biologic, 56
biological, 22, 26, 29, 35, 36, 39
biology, 19, 85, 92
biopsies, 25
biosynthesis, 29
bisulfite treatment-specific PCR, 4
bladder, 29, 36, 49, 84
bladder cancer, 49, 84
blocks, 29
blood, 45
blot, 59
bone, 35, 61, 76, 83
borderline, 29
brain, 23, 48
BRCA, 45
BRCA1, v, vii, 1, 6, 9, 10, 11, 14, 27, 44, 47,
    48, 59, 64, 73, 79, 80, 81, 88, 91, 92, 95,
    99, 101
BRCA1-associated genome surveillance
    complex (BASC), 9
BRCA2, v, vii, 1, 6, 9, 10, 11, 13, 27, 47, 64,
    73, 79, 80, 88, 91, 99
breast carcinoma, 9, 17, 20, 21, 31, 38, 39, 40,
    42, 43, 45, 48, 51, 53, 59, 60, 61, 62, 64,
    65, 71, 74, 77, 78, 80, 82, 83, 84, 85, 87,
    92, 94, 95, 96, 100, 101
Breast Information Core, 9
bypass, 57

C

cadherin (s), 72, 73, 74, 76, 86, 90, 93
calcium, 11, 15, 50
cancer cells, 1, 7, 15, 16, 17, 19, 22, 31, 32,
    33, 35, 36, 37, 42, 43, 53, 56, 57, 58, 59,
    61, 62, 65, 73, 75, 76, 79, 81, 83, 86, 95,
    100, 101
cancer progression, 30, 34, 60, 62, 63, 72, 74,
    83, 84, 87, 91
carbazole, 7
carboxyl, 59
carcinogenesis, 19, 26, 27, 28, 47, 65, 90
carcinogens, 5, 24
carcinoma (s), 9, 15, 17, 20, 21, 23, 30, 31,
    33, 34, 38, 39, 40, 41, 42, 43, 45, 48, 49,
    50, 51, 53, 57, 58, 59, 60, 61, 62, 64, 65,
    71, 74, 76, 77, 78, 79, 80, 82, 83, 84, 85,
    86, 87, 90, 92, 94, 95, 96, 98, 100, 101, 102
cargo, 58
carrier, 15
caspase, 31, 63, 73
cation, 12
CBF, 72
CDK2, 45
CDK4, 13
cDNA, 22, 37, 81
cell, vii, 1, 5, 6, 7, 10, 13, 15, 16, 17, 18, 19,
    20, 21, 22, 23, 24, 25, 26, 27, 28, 29, 30,
    32, 33, 34, 35, 36, 37, 38, 39, 40, 41, 42,
    43, 45, 46, 47, 48, 49, 50, 51, 52, 53, 54,
    55, 56, 58, 59, 60, 61, 62, 63, 64, 65, 67,
    73, 74, 76, 78, 79, 80, 82, 83, 88, 90, 92,
    94, 95, 96, 97, 98, 99, 101, 102
cell adhesion, 19, 43, 50
cell cycle, vii, 5, 10, 19, 22, 23, 29, 36, 38, 46,
    47, 49, 54, 55, 62, 64, 80, 88
cell death, 1, 7, 13, 47, 59, 63, 79, 83, 102
cell fate, 5

cell growth, 1, 35, 36, 39, 42, 47, 50, 62, 63, 82, 97, 98, 101, 102
cell line (s), 6, 15, 16, 17, 18, 19, 20, 21, 22, 23, 24, 26, 27, 28, 29, 30, 33, 34, 35, 36, 37, 38, 41, 42, 43, 45, 46, 47, 48, 50, 52, 53, 54, 56, 58, 59, 60, 61, 62, 63, 65, 73, 76, 78, 82, 90, 92, 94, 95, 98, 99
cell membranes, 51
centromeric, 59
centrosome, 10
cervical, 23, 48, 94
cervical cancer, 48
cervical carcinoma, 94
cervix, 6
channels, 56, 59
CHEK2, 1, 6, 15, 27, 43, 64, 76, 88, 89, 93, 95, 99
chemical, 7, 24
chemoattractant, 61
chemoprevention, 84
chemopreventive, 26
chemotherapeutic agent, 41
chemotherapeutic drugs, 7
chemotherapy, 7
chicken, 12
chloride, 11, 15, 56, 80
chromatid, 10
chromatin, 10, 15, 16, 21, 50, 51, 62, 67, 95
chromosomal abnormalities, 53
chromosome (s), 10, 12, 14, 15, 16, 17, 19, 20, 21, 23, 25, 31, 32, 33, 35, 37, 42, 43, 44, 45, 47, 48, 54, 55, 56, 58, 59, 63, 65, 71, 72, 74, 75, 77, 78, 79, 80, 81, 82, 83, 84, 85, 86, 87, 89, 90, 92, 93, 94, 96, 97, 98, 99, 100, 101, 102
cisplatin, 7
classes, 10, 44
classical, 3, 53
classification, 80
classified, 27
clinical, 7, 60, 72, 73, 82, 92, 97
clinicopathologic, 46
clone (s), 23, 42, 83
cloning, 20, 40, 43, 58, 81, 88
codes, 42

coding, 6, 17, 21, 27, 31, 48, 55, 59, 97
codon (s), 6, 37, 45, 50
coil, 14, 16, 36
Collaboration, 92
colocalization, 10
colon, 23, 29, 33, 36, 56
colorectal, 12, 15, 30, 61, 72, 74, 82, 83, 93, 97
colorectal cancer, 12, 30, 72, 74, 97
complement, 12
complementary DNA, 78
components, 10, 36, 40, 42, 63
compounds, 7, 17
consensus, 91
conservation, 36
control, vii, 7, 19, 28, 29, 33, 35, 36, 38, 44, 45, 47, 49, 55, 56
conversion, ix, 10
correlation (s), 23, 26, 34, 37, 40, 41, 46, 54, 79, 91
coupling, 38
Cowden syndrome, 6
CpG islands, 16, 31
cues, 27
culture, 50
cyclin D1, 15, 38
cyclin-dependent kinase inhibitor, 49, 92
cyclooxygenase, 28, 74, 92
cyclooxygenase-2 (COX-2), 28, 92
Cystatin, 13, 71
cysteine proteases, 42
cytogenetic (s), 20, 87, 90, 97
cytokeratins, 53
cytokinesis, 39
cytology, 98
cytoplasm, 17, 18, 58, 64
cytoskeleton, 34, 35, 59, 65, 95, 98
cytosol, 36
cytotoxic, 5, 41

D

daughter cells, 3
death, 1, 7, 13, 47, 63, 79, 83, 102
defects, 64

deficiency, 21
definition, vii, 91
degradation, 5, 10, 29, 32, 54, 58
degrading, 42
dehydrogenase, 12, 29, 100
deletions, 1, 19, 21, 22, 23, 29, 35, 38, 39, 56, 59, 61, 78, 94, 96
delivery, 56, 58
density, 3, 81
deposits, 39
deprivation, 56
dermal, 49
detection, 33, 47
developmental disorder, 48
diabetes mellitus, 31
differentiation, 1, 21, 32, 38, 92
Discovery, 94, 100
disease free survival, 16, 53
disease progression, 60
diseases, 49
disorder, 30, 62
distal, 43, 85, 93
distribution, 36
diversity, 83
DLC, 79, 91, 101
DNA, vii, 5, 6, 7, 9, 10, 13, 17, 19, 20, 24, 25, 27, 29, 34, 36, 37, 41, 42, 43, 47, 55, 57, 59, 62, 64, 65, 67, 74, 78, 81, 91, 92, 95, 99, 101
DNA damage, 9, 20, 27, 36, 47, 57, 64, 91
DNA repair, vii, 5, 6, 7, 9, 10, 41, 47, 64, 67, 95
double-strand breaks (DSB), ix, 10, 17, 27, 43, 64
down-regulation, 39, 41, 46, 54, 95
DPP, 15
Drosophila, 11, 12, 13, 15, 75
drug-induced, 22
drugs, 5, 7
duration, 37

E

E. coli, 15, 72
E-cadherin, 72, 73, 74, 76, 86, 93

EGFR, 21
elongation, 58, 89
embryonic, 24, 42, 74, 98, 101
embryonic development, 74, 101
encoding, 62, 76, 81
endometrium, 95
enzyme (s), 29, 32, 41, 62
epidemiological, 44
epigenetic, 1, 15, 16, 21, 28, 29, 31, 33, 37, 43, 50, 57, 58, 74, 81, 88, 95
epigenetic mechanism, 16, 34, 37
epigenetic silencing, 29, 33, 43, 58, 88
epithelia, 95
epithelial cells, 1, 17, 18, 30, 32, 37, 42, 49, 53, 60, 78
epithelial ovarian cancer, 88
epithelial tumours, 73
epithelium, 15, 18, 25, 41, 43, 54, 57, 61
Escherichia coli, 47
esophageal, 46, 82
estrogen, 20, 22, 25, 32, 40, 46, 60, 61, 76, 86, 95, 99
estrogen receptor-positive breast cancer, 95
eukaryotes, 10
eukaryotic cell, 46
European, 72, 81, 82, 91
evidence, 6, 17, 18, 20, 26, 33, 39, 43, 44, 47, 54, 60, 80, 88, 90, 95
evolution, 79
evolutionary, 36
excision, ix, 10
exclusion, 75, 93
execution, 54
exogenous, 22
exons, 26, 27, 30, 38
extinction, 43
extracellular matrix, 33, 42, 63, 81

F

familial, vii, 6, 20, 27, 30, 44, 47, 48, 64, 78, 80, 90, 98, 100
familial aggregation, 27
family, 9, 11, 12, 15, 16, 24, 25, 27, 36, 39, 47, 48, 55, 60, 62, 63, 73, 75, 76, 93

family history, 9, 48
FANCD1, 13
fatty acid (s), 17
F-box, 14, 54
fibroblasts, 24
fidelity, 44, 91, 99
follicle, 40
fragile site, 12, 20, 53
frameshift mutation, 19, 50, 88

G

gall bladder, 49
gamma-aminobutyric acid (GABA), 14, 56, 98
gastric, 18, 31, 36, 53, 78, 83, 85, 89, 98
gastrointestinal, 62
gene (s), ix, 1, 3, 6, 7, 10, 11, 12, 13, 14, 15, 16, 17, 18, 19, 20, 21, 22, 23, 24, 25, 26, 27, 28, 30, 31, 32, 33, 34, 35, 36, 37, 38, 39, 41, 42, 43, 44, 45, 46, 47, 48, 50, 51, 52, 53, 54, 55, 56, 57, 58, 60, 61, 62, 64, 65, 67, 71, 72, 73, 74, 75, 76, 77, 78, 79, 80, 81, 82, 83, 84, 85, 86, 87, 88, 89, 90, 91, 92, 93, 94, 95, 96, 97, 98, 99, 100, 101, 102
gene amplification, 1
gene conversion, ix
gene expression, 26, 43, 54, 62, 76, 80, 81, 86, 91, 95
gene promoter, 1, 3, 4, 30, 72, 90, 98
gene silencing, 15, 34, 43, 50, 52
genetic (s), vii, 1, 3, 6, 7, 16, 21, 35, 38, 40, 46, 47, 50, 51, 57, 74, 83, 85, 87, 89, 93, 99, 100
genetic alteration, vii, 46, 57, 93, 100
genetic disease, 1
genetic diversity, 83
genetic instability, 7
genome, 6, 9, 20, 81, 86, 88
genomic, 3, 27, 34, 35, 36, 37, 38, 43, 50, 53, 59, 62, 71, 74, 78, 82, 86, 89, 91, 93, 100
genomic instability, 37, 43
genotoxic, 5
genotype, 85

germ line, 76
glycoprotein, 50
glycosylation, 5
grading, 48, 87
growth, 1, 7, 11, 12, 15, 18, 22, 23, 24, 27, 29, 31, 32, 33, 34, 35, 36, 38, 39, 41, 42, 43, 47, 50, 53, 55, 56, 58, 60, 62, 63, 67, 73, 75, 76, 79, 81, 82, 83, 84, 86, 87, 89, 91, 97, 98, 99, 101, 102
growth factor (s), 12, 29, 32, 41, 60, 75, 76, 79, 84, 87, 89, 97, 102
growth rate, 31, 56
guanine, 41
guidance, 11, 24, 27, 101

H

hair follicle, 40
haploinsufficiency, 3
heart, 48
hematologic, 41
hematoma, 62
hepatocellular carcinoma, 59, 83, 102
hereditary, vii, 1, 6, 9, 12, 27, 64, 85
heterodimer, 49
heterogeneity, 83
heterozygosity, ix, 3, 13, 57, 58, 64, 71, 74, 75, 77, 79, 83, 84, 85, 86, 87, 88, 89, 91, 92, 93, 100
high risk, 27, 40, 47, 48, 77, 79
high-level, 30
histidine, 12, 20, 94
histological, 24, 48, 62, 86, 87
histone, 16, 18, 25, 29, 31, 34, 76, 83, 90
homolog, 11, 12, 13, 14, 15, 55
homology, ix, 10, 15, 19, 35
homology-directed recombination, ix, 10
Honda, 101
hormone, 20, 50
hot spots, 6
human (s), 5, 6, 7, 16, 17, 18, 19, 20, 21, 22, 23, 24, 25, 26, 28, 31, 32, 33, 34, 35, 36, 37, 38, 39, 43, 44, 45, 46, 47, 56, 57, 58, 59, 60, 61, 62, 64, 65, 71, 72, 74, 75, 76, 77, 78, 79, 80, 81, 82, 83, 84, 85, 86, 87,

88, 89, 91, 92, 93, 94, 95, 96, 97, 99, 100, 101, 102
human genome, 20
hybridization, 3, 74, 78, 86, 89, 100
hydrogen, 15
hydrophobic, 17
hypermethylation, 3, 15, 18, 20, 22, 24, 26, 28, 32, 34, 37, 38, 39, 40, 43, 45, 46, 51, 57, 71, 73, 77, 85, 94, 96, 100
hyper-mutable, 6
hyperplasia, 25
hypothesis, 3, 19, 28, 52, 74
hypoxia, 5

I

identification, 37, 56, 57, 83, 85, 91
IGF-I, 81
immunocompromised, 34
immunodeficient, 33
immunoglobulin, 12
immunohistochemical, 49
immunohistochemistry, 25
immunoreactivity, 17
imprinting, 50, 60
in situ, 32, 33, 48, 51, 77, 98
in vitro, 7, 17, 22, 23, 29, 31, 32, 34, 45, 83
in vivo, 7, 22, 23, 29, 32, 36, 38, 45, 83, 101
inactivated genes, 3
inactive, 56
incidence, 6, 38, 58, 59, 100
index case, 27
indication, 85
induction, 7, 10, 26, 73, 97
infection, 28
inheritance, 40
inherited, 1, 9, 49, 64, 73, 89
inhibition, 16, 22, 24, 32, 34, 35, 36, 45, 47, 84, 86, 90
inhibitor, 11, 13, 32, 42, 49, 59, 81, 90, 91, 92, 98
inhibitory, 23, 56
inhibitory effect, 98
initiation, 40
inositol, 39

insertion, 52
instability, 7, 21, 37, 43, 92, 93
instructors, 73
insulation, 50
insulin, 32, 41, 49, 75, 89
insulin signaling, 49
insulin-like growth factor (IGF), 32, 41, 75, 81, 89
integrity, 27, 91
intensity, 51
interaction (s), 1, 5, 6, 7, 10, 25, 40, 47, 56, 59, 60, 81
interference, 24, 56
international, 99
International Agency for Research on Cancer, 6
interval, 81, 101
inversion, 92
Investigations, 83, 91, 92
ion channels, 59
ion transport, 59, 60
ionizing radiation, 27, 91
irradiation, 5
irreversible, 5
island, 19, 22, 28, 57, 75
isomerization, 5

J

Japan, 101
Japanese, 83, 100
JNK, 15

K

kidney (s), 20, 21, 22, 48, 65, 82
kinase (s), 13, 14, 15, 19, 25, 32, 38, 39, 4, 49, 55, 60, 62, 64, 75, 79, 80, 89, 92, 97, 99
kinase activity, 32, 62
King, 9, 10, 80, 99
knockout, 3

L

large-scale, 35
latency, 33
lead, 42, 47, 67
lesions, 7, 25, 26, 38, 49, 59, 61, 82, 87
leucine, 14, 82
lifespan, 24
Li-Fraumeni-like syndrome, 6
ligand, 56
likelihood, 37
linear, 10
linkage, 58
links, 98
linoleic acid, 99
lipid (s), 17, 39
liver cancer, 13, 28, 63, 65
localization, 36, 39, 77
location, 19, 63
locus, 5, 16, 30, 31, 32, 33, 38, 40, 42, 45, 54, 57, 59, 60, 61, 75, 78, 79, 83, 84, 87, 89, 93, 94, 101
loss of heterozygosity (LOH), vii, ix, 3, 5, 9, 16, 17, 18, 19, 20, 21, 23, 24, 25, 26, 27, 29, 30, 31, 32, 33, 35, 36, 40, 41, 42, 43, 44, 45, 46, 48, 49, 51, 52, 53, 54, 55, 56, 57, 59, 60, 61, 62, 63, 64, 65, 71, 74, 79, 83, 84, 87, 88, 91, 92, 93, 100
losses, 5, 19, 57, 65, 81, 87, 94
lung, 6, 13, 19, 20, 21, 22, 23, 24, 29, 30, 49, 59, 60, 71, 73, 74, 75, 79, 84, 85, 89, 90, 93, 94, 96, 97, 98
lung cancer, 13, 19, 20, 21, 22, 23, 24, 85, 89, 90, 93, 96, 97
lymph, 32, 40, 46, 53, 62, 94, 99
lymph node, 32, 40, 46, 53, 62, 94
lymphoma (s), 23, 63, 59
lysine, 18
lysosomal enzymes, 32
lysosome, 58

M

machinery, 62

maintenance, 24, 27
malignancy, 45
malignant, 1, 10, 25, 39, 57, 73, 75, 84, 95
malignant cells, 39
malignant growth, 75
malignant mesothelioma, 84
malignant tumors, 57
mammalian cells, 17, 24
mammoplasty, 34
MAPK, 14
mapping, 57, 75, 93, 94, 96, 99
mass spectrometry, 97
maternal, 16
matrix, 15, 33, 42, 63, 81
matrix metalloproteinase, 33
MCC, 87
MDA, 15, 29, 33, 42, 49, 53, 56, 65
median, 63
mediators, 36
membranes, 40, 51, 58
memory, 69
meningioma, 79
mental retardation, 48
mesenchymal, 61, 76
messenger RNA, 81
metabolism, 17
metalloproteinases, 33
metastasis, 15, 32, 35, 37, 38, 40, 46, 49, 53, 61, 62, 76, 79, 83, 94, 99
metastatic, 34, 48, 100
methylated, vii, 3, 16, 26, 28, 30, 41, 49, 51, 57
methylation, 1, 4, 5, 16, 18, 19, 22, 24, 25, 26, 28, 29, 30, 31, 33, 34, 36, 39, 41, 42, 43, 46, 47, 49, 50, 51, 52, 54, 55, 56, 57, 60, 63, 64, 71, 72, 75, 76, 78, 79, 81, 82, 83, 84, 86, 90, 92, 98
methylation-specific PCR (MSP), 4
MGMT, 13, 41
mice, 5, 7, 17, 18, 22, 23, 24, 29, 31, 32, 33, 34, 38, 42, 56, 59, 62, 79, 89
microarray, 3, 35, 78, 86
microenvironment, 33
microtubule, 5, 36
migration, 19, 34, 43

minority, 1
MIRA-1, 7
mitochondria, 17
mitogen, 12, 14, 32, 55, 97
mitogen-activated protein kinase, 55, 97
mitogenic, 29, 31, 95
mitosis, 19, 36, 39, 82
mitotic, 7
modeling, 33
molecular mechanisms, 20
molecules, 10, 59
morphology, 17
mortality, 49
mouse model, 37
mRNA, 18, 21, 23, 25, 29, 32, 33, 34, 37, 38, 40, 45, 46, 48, 49, 52, 53, 56, 64, 65, 92, 96
multivariate, 20
mutagenesis, 89
mutant (s), 6, 7, 10, 24, 25, 30, 44, 48, 64, 79
mutation (s), vii, 1, 3, 4, 6, 7, 9, 10, 15, 16, 17, 18, 19, 21, 22, 23, 24, 25, 26, 27, 29, 30, 31, 32, 33, 34, 35, 38, 39, 40, 41, 42, 43, 44, 45, 46, 47, 48, 50, 51, 52, 53, 54, 55, 56, 57, 58, 59, 60, 61, 62, 64, 65, 72, 73, 75, 76, 81, 82, 83, 84, 87, 88, 89, 91, 92, 95, 96, 97, 99, 100
MYC, 46
myeloid, 14
myosin, 14

N

Na^+, 59, 75
National Academy of Sciences, 74, 80, 82, 84, 87, 97, 101, 102
neddylation, 5
negative regulatory, 39
negative selection, 19
negativity, 32, 46
neoplasia (s), 46, 53
neoplasm (s), 31, 34, 39, 49, 81
neoplastic, 26, 59, 60
network, 10, 35, 83
neural crest, 65
neuroblastoma, 23

neuroendocrine, 79
Neurofibromatosis, 15
neurotransmission, 56
neurotransmitter, 56
New York, 79, 85, 101
Nielsen, 95
nodules, 49
non-homologous end joining (NHEJ), ix, 10, 44, 64
nonsense mutation, 72
normal, 1, 5, 7, 15, 16, 18, 20, 24, 25, 26, 28, 29, 34, 35, 37, 38, 41, 43, 45, 46, 47, 49, 54, 55, 56, 57, 63, 64, 83, 92, 95
nuclear, 5, 9, 22, 39, 41, 43, 95
nucleolus, 63
nucleotide sequence, 100
nucleotide-excision repair (NER), ix, 10
nucleus, 36, 39

O

observations, 19, 50
oligonucleotide, 3, 81, 86
Oncogene (s), 1, 5, 24, 39, 71, 72, 73, 74, 75, 76, 78, 80, 81, 82, 83, 85, 86, 87, 88, 89, 91, 93, 94, oncogenes
oncogenesis, 55, 86
Oncology, 82, 83, 84, 88, 91, 92, 96, 97, 99, 100
oncoproteins, 46
oral, 23
organ, 1, 35
organelles, 17, 58
organization, 34, 71, 76, 82
orientation, 55
ovarian, 9, 16, 27, 28, 29, 32, 33, 49, 58, 59, 71, 73, 77, 80, 85, 88, 90, 97, 99, 101
ovarian cancer (s), 16, 27, 29, 58, 73, 77, 80, 85, 88, 99, 101
ovary, 36
oxidation, 17

P

pairing, 47
pancreatic, 15, 16, 56, 61, 96, 98
pancreatic cancer, 15, 16
paternal, 16
pathogenesis, 62, 64
pathology, 85
pathways, 1, 7, 10, 16, 38, 47, 51, 55, 67, 95
patients, 20, 30, 38, 41, 48, 49, 53, 64, 87, 88
PCR, 4, 49, 94
PDZ domains, 59
penetrance, 88
Peutz-Jeghers syndrome, 6
phagocytosis, 38
phenotype (s), 7, 35, 44, 46, 53, 73, 79, 83, 85, 96
phosphate, 12, 32, 39, 75, 89
phosphoprotein, 12
phosphorylates, 90
phosphorylation, 5, 44
physical interaction, 6
physiological, 16, 24, 35, 39
PI3K, 39
plasma membrane, 17, 39
plastic, 53
play, 10, 17, 22, 28, 31, 59, 60, 61, 65
point mutation, vii, 1, 3, 18, 30, 31, 32, 40, 41, 42, 58, 60, 61, 89
poisons, 7
polymerase chain reaction, 41
polymorphism (s), 4, 52, 54, 55
polypeptide (s), 12, 36
poor, 21, 32, 33, 41, 43, 72, 76, 77, 81, 84, 88
population, 45, 55, 64, 80
postoperative, 77, 81
pre-existing, 57
primary tumor, 29, 34, 36, 41, 50, 52, 54, 73
pro-apoptotic protein, 35
progesterone, 20, 24, 32, 46
prognosis, 32, 33, 41, 43, 52, 53, 77, 79, 81, 84, 88, 91, 94, 98
prognostic marker, 21, 72
program, 83
progressive, 25

proliferation, vii, 7, 16, 17, 21, 24, 28, 29, 34, 38, 41, 42, 43, 46, 50, 53, 56, 59, 74, 98, 101
promote, 28, 99
promoter, 1, 3, 4, 7, 15, 18, 19, 22, 24, 26, 28, 29, 30, 32, 33, 34, 37, 39, 40, 41, 43, 45, 46, 47, 49, 50, 51, 52, 54, 56, 57, 60, 63, 71, 72, 73, 75, 76, 77, 82, 85, 86, 90, 95, 96, 98
promoter region, 15, 22, 24, 32, 43, 46, 47, 51, 73, 75
proposition, 32
prostaglandin (s), 29, 74
prostate, 3, 19, 23, 33, 36, 48, 50, 52, 55, 59, 74, 78, 81, 84, 98
prostate cancer, 3, 33, 48, 52, 59, 78, 81, 84, 98
proteases, 42
protein (s), 4, 5, 6, 7, 9, 10, 11, 12, 13, 14, 15, 16, 17, 18, 19, 20, 21, 22, 23, 24, 25, 27, 28, 29, 31, 33, 34, 35, 36, 37, 38, 39, 40, 41, 42, 43, 44, 47, 48, 49, 51, 53, 54, 55, 56, 58, 59, 60, 62, 63, 64, 65, 72, 73, 75, 76, 77, 79, 82, 84, 85, 86, 89, 90, 91, 95, 98, 99, 101, 102
protein function, 99
protein kinases, 43, 55
protein structure, 47
proximal, 36, 43, 61
PTEN, 1, 3, 6, 13, 27, 39, 40, 76, 77, 78, 79, 90, 92

R

radiation, 27, 91
Raman, 77
range, 27, 48, 65
RAS, 11, 22, 45, 46, 75
rat, 16
RB1, 14, 38, 46, 80
reading, 12, 14, 17, 38, 55
real-time, 94
receptor-positive, 22, 95
receptors, 20, 24, 26, 27, 53, 56, 59, 73, 98
recombination, ix, 10, 14, 17, 47, 67, 87, 91

reconcile, 48
recurrence, 49, 79, 81
reduction, 24, 25, 42, 54, 61
regulation, 1, 10, 15, 16, 27, 29, 34, 36, 39,
    41, 46, 49, 50, 54, 56, 62, 78, 81, 90, 92,
    95, 96, 101
regulators, 18, 43, 49
reinforcement, 10
relationship (s), 38, 51, 53, 85, 93, 98
relatives, 44
relevance, 24, 92
remodeling, 10, 21, 62, 67, 81
renal, 15, 23, 31, 94, 96
renal cell carcinoma, 23, 96
repair, ix, 5, 6, 7, 9, 10, 17, 23, 41, 43, 47, 64,
    67, 95, 101
replication, 91
repression, 50, 57
repressor, 36, 39, 57, 91, 99
research, 9
residues, 6
resistance, 7, 24, 28, 57
resolution, 86, 87, 89, 100
responsiveness, 90
restoration, 7, 34, 47
retardation, 31, 48
retention, 95
retinoblastoma, 11, 14, 23, 84
retinoic acid receptor, 26, 95
retinoids, 26
reversible, 5, 18, 52
Rho, 13, 34, 67
risk, 9, 20, 25, 27, 40, 42, 44, 45, 47, 48, 62,
    63, 64, 77, 78, 79
risk factors, 9
RNA, 12, 22, 24, 35, 37, 56, 72, 81

S

sample, 51, 65
sarcomas, 7, 32
scaffold, 6, 81
scalp, 49
sclerosis, 13, 14, 48, 92
search, 83

secretion, 16, 73
seizures, 48
senescence, 5, 12, 23, 24, 53, 83, 84, 89
sensing, 10
sensors, 36
sequencing, 3, 48
series, 1, 9, 17, 25, 32, 41, 45, 48, 65
serine, 15, 25, 62, 63
serum, 56
signal transduction, vii, 1, 29, 55, 59
signaling, vii, 15, 19, 22, 23, 25, 31, 38, 39,
    49, 60, 67, 79, 84
signaling pathway (s), 25, 30, 31, 49, 67
signals, 5, 56
single strand chain polymorphism, 4
single-strand annealing (SSA), ix, 10
sites, 5, 20, 50, 53, 61, 62
skin, 19, 48
SNP, 3, 97
sodium, 15
soft tissue sarcomas, 32
solid tumors, 31, 41, 57
somatic cell (s), 46, 49
somatic mutations, 15, 45, 62, 65
species, 38
specificity, 78
spectrum, 58
speculation, 38
S-phase, 20
spindle, 7
spleen, 99
sporadic, 9, 15, 17, 20, 31, 40, 46, 48, 49, 54,
    56, 57, 59, 61, 62, 64, 71, 77, 80, 89, 93,
    95, 96, 97, 100
squamous cell carcinoma, 82
stages, 83
steroid hormone, 21
STK11, 1, 6, 15, 62, 92
stress, 5, 56
stromal, 32, 49
structural protein, 60
substitution, 65
substrates, 54
sumoylation, 5
Sun, 52, 86, 96

suppression, 7, 13, 19, 24, 26, 31, 33, 34, 36, 42, 45, 56, 73, 81, 86, 99, 100

suppressor (s), vii, ix, 1, 12, 13, 14, 17, 18, 19, 22, 26, 27, 29, 33, 35, 38, 39, 41, 48, 50, 53, 54, 56, 58, 59, 60, 63, 64, 67, 71, 72, 73, 74, 75, 76, 77, 78, 79, 80, 81, 82, 84, 85, 86, 87, 88, 89, 90, 91, 92, 93, 94, 95, 96, 97, 98, 99, 100, 101, 102

surveillance, 9

survival, 6, 16, 20, 37, 38, 42, 53, 61, 62, 67, 82, 98

susceptibility, 9, 13, 20, 22, 27, 34, 40, 44, 56, 59, 62, 64, 71, 81, 88, 89, 92, 93, 95, 97

susceptibility genes, 27, 97

syndrome, 6, 13, 40, 42, 43, 48, 62, 100

synthesis, 17, 29

systems, 41

T

T cell, 63

targets, 39

telangiectasia, 12, 13, 43, 44, 92, 99

telomerase, 36, 46

testicular cancer, 100

testis, 56

theory, 7

threonine, 15, 25, 62

thyroid, 40

time, 94

Timmer, 72

tissue, 17, 26, 32, 34, 36, 38, 45, 54, 56, 57, 63, 95

TNF-alpha, 22

toxins, 58

Toyota, 84

TP53, vii, 1, 5, 6, 7, 11, 14, 27, 47, 57, 58, 89, 93

transcript, 11, 12, 26, 30, 36, 49, 91

transcription, 5, 10, 11, 14, 16, 18, 26, 31, 39, 41, 50, 51, 52, 57, 62, 78, 95

transcription factor (s), 5, 11, 14, 31, 41, 50, 51, 52, 78

transcriptional, 7, 10, 31, 37, 39, 41, 51, 52, 57, 62, 91

transcripts, 26, 35, 36, 59

transducer, 64

transduction, 1, 29, 47, 55, 59

transfection, 56

transfer, 42

transformation, 1, 10, 12, 24, 34

transforming growth factor (TGF), 18, 24, 25, 41, 60, 61, 67, 76, 79, 84, 87, 95, 97, 102

transgenic, 5, 79

transition, 48, 61, 76

translation, 40

translocation (s), 1, 14, 39, 47

transmembrane, 16, 25, 63

transmission, 9

transport, 17, 60

trend, 30, 54

trichostatin A, 65

Tuberous sclerosis complex (TSC), 48, 49, 82, 92

tubular, 61

tumor, vii, ix, 1, 3, 5, 7, 12, 13, 14, 16, 17, 18, 19, 21, 22, 23, 24, 25, 26, 27, 28, 29, 30, 31, 32, 33, 34, 35, 36, 37, 38, 39, 41, 42, 43, 44, 45, 46, 48, 49, 50, 52, 53, 54, 55, 56, 58, 59, 60, 61, 62, 63, 64, 65, 67, 71, 72, 73, 74, 75, 76, 77, 78, 79, 80, 82, 83, 84, 85, 86, 87, 88, 89, 90, 91, 92, 93, 94, 95, 96, 97, 98, 99, 100, 101, 102

tumor cells, 22, 28, 37, 56, 63, 79, 91

tumor growth, 16, 31, 38, 43, 56, 61, 83, 86

tumor metastasis, 35

tumor progression, 3, 16, 37, 82

tumor suppressor gene (TSG) (s), vii, ix, 1, 3, 5, 9, 11, 15, 16, 17, 18, 19, 20, 21, 23, 24, 25, 26, 28, 29, 30, 31, 32, 33, 34, 37, 40, 41, 42, 44, 45, 46, 48, 50, 52, 53, 54, 55, 56, 58, 57, 59, 60, 61, 62, 63, 64, 65, 67, 71, 73, 74, 75, 76, 77, 78, 80, 82, 84, 85, 86, 87, 88, 89, 90, 91, 92, 93, 94, 96, 97, 98, 100, 101

tumorigenesis, 3, 7, 16, 18, 20, 25, 28, 39, 41, 47, 58, 64, 65, 74, 86, 91, 92, 99

tumorigenic, 38, 46, 83

tumors, 1, 5, 6, 7, 9, 15, 16, 17, 19, 20, 21, 22, 23, 24, 25, 26, 27, 28, 29, 30, 31, 32, 33,

34, 35, 36, 37, 38, 40, 41, 42, 43, 44, 45,
46, 48, 49, 50, 51, 52, 53, 54, 55, 56, 57,
58, 59, 60, 61, 62, 64, 65, 72, 73, 75, 79,
82, 84, 85, 86, 91, 92, 93, 98
tumour (s), 34, 71, 73, 74, 75, 77, 78, 79, 84,
85, 92, 95, 97, 98
tumour suppressor genes, 77, 84, 97
two-hit, 3, 28, 52, 53, 74
tyrosine, 11, 13, 20, 38, 75, 89, 99

U

ubiquitin, 5, 10, 58
ubiquitinate, 7
undifferentiated, 61
United States, 74, 80, 82, 84, 87, 97, 101, 102
users, 89

V

variation, 48, 55, 64, 86
vehicles, 17

W

Wales, 57, 98
warts, 12, 88
Washington, 87
wild type, 95
wild-type allele, 62
Wnt signaling, 30
women, 25, 64

X

xenograft (s), 7, 16, 31, 37, 56

Y

yeast, 15, 48, 62

Z

zinc, 11, 14, 18, 37, 50, 78